CRASH COURSE
Immunology and Haematology

SECOND EDITION

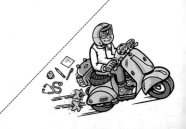

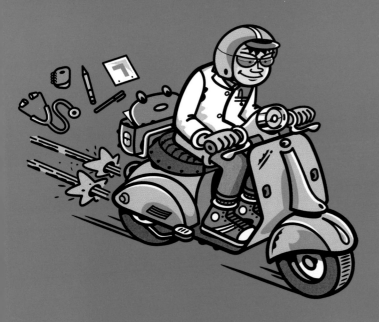

Series editor
Daniel Horton-Szar
BSc (Hons), MBBS (Hons)
GP Registrar
Northgate Medical Practice
Canterbury
Kent

Faculty advisors
Matthew Helbert
MRCP MRCPath PhD
Consultant Immunologist
Department of Immunology
St Mary's Hospital
Oxford Road
Manchester

John Amess
MB FRCP FRCPath
Consultant Haematologist
Department of Haematology
St Bartholomew's Hospital
West Smithfield
London

Immunology and Haematology

SECOND EDITION

James Griffin

BSc (Hons)
5th Year medical student
Centre for Medical Education
St Michael's Hill
Bristol

First edition authors
Saimah Arif, Arjmand Mufti

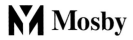

Edinburgh • London • New York • Oxford • Philadelphia • St Louis • Sydney • Toronto 2003

MOSBY
An imprint of Elsevier Limited

Commissioning editor	Alex Stibbe
Project Manager	Frances Affleck
Project Development Manager	Duncan Fraser
Designer	Andy Chapman
Cover Design	Kevin Faerber
Illustration Manager	Mick Ruddy

First edition © 1998, Mosby International Ltd
This edition © 2003, Elsevier Ltd

First edition 1998
Second edition 2003
   Reprinted 2003, 2004, 2005, 2006

ISBN 0723432929

British Library Cataloguing in Publication Data
A catalogue record for this book is available from the British Library

Library of Congress Cataloguing in Publication Data
A catalogue record for this book is available from the Library of Congress

Note
Medical knowledge is constantly changing. As new information becomes available,
changes in treatment, procedures, equipment and the use of drugs become
necessary. The author, editors and the publishers have taken care to ensure that the
information given in this text is accurate and up to date. However, readers are
strongly advised to confirm that the information, especially with regard to drug
usage, complies with the latest legislation and standards of practice.

ELSEVIER
your s urce for books,
journals and multimedia
in the health sciences
www.elsevierhealth.com

Working together to grow
libraries in developing countries
www.elsevier.com | www.bookaid.org | www.sabre.org
ELSEVIER   BOOK AID International   Sabre Foundation

The
publisher's
policy is to use
**paper manufactured
from sustainable forests**

Typeset by SNP Best-set Typesetter Ltd , Hong Kong
Printed in China

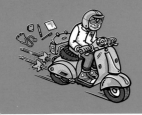

Preface

When fellow medical students found out that I was writing this book, a large number asked 'Great, will it be out in time for finals?' Many medical students find it difficult to understand immunological and haematological principles and to remember the necessary facts. They honestly aren't too difficult to learn but they are very important. Aspects of immunology and haematology crop up again and again in many different fields of medicine—these subjects, however, often seem to be poorly taught.

In *Crash Course: Immunology and Haematology* I've tried to cover as much ground as possible so, by the time your exams come around, you should have, at least, a basic grasp of most immunological and haematological principles. Basic science and clinical information have been combined to place the science into the context of clinical practice. I hope I have succeeded and that you enjoy using this book.

James Griffin

In the six years since the first editions were published, there have been many changes in medicine, and in the way it is taught. These second editions have been largely rewritten to take these changes into account, and keep Crash Course up to date for the twenty-first century. New material has been added to include recent research and all pharmacological and disease management information has been updated in line with current best practice. We've listened to feedback from hundreds of students who have been using Crash Course and have improved the structure and layout of the books accordingly: pathology material has been closely integrated with the relevant basic medical science; there are more MCQs and the clarity of text and figures is better than ever.

The principles on which we developed the series remain the same, however. Medicine is a huge subject, and the last thing a student needs when exams are looming is to waste time assembling information from different sources, and wading through pages of irrelevant detail. As before, Crash Course brings you all the information you need, in compact, manageable volumes that integrate basic medical science with clinical practice. We still tread the fine line between producing clear, concise text and providing enough detail for those aiming at distinction. The series is still written by medical students with recent exam experience, and checked for accuracy by senior faculty members from across the UK.

I wish you the best of luck in your future careers!

Dr Dan Horton-Szar
Series Editor (Basic Medical Sciences)

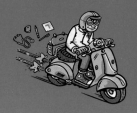

Acknowledgements

The author would like to thank several people for their help during the writing and production of this book: Dan Horton Szar, Matthew Helbert and John Amess for their input, gratefully received; and the staff at Elsevier Science without whose expertise, useful advice and help throughout the writing process, the book would not look like it does today.

Figure acknowledgement

Figs 1.2 and 2.5 adapted with permission from C Janeway. Immunobiology, 4th edition. Churchill Livingston, 1999

Figs 1.19, 1.25, 1.30, 1.31, 1.35, 1.37, 2.18, 2.26 and 3.4, adapted with permission from I Roitt, D Male and I Brostoff. Immunology, 4th edition. Mosby, 1996

Figs 2.5, 4.1 and 4.14, taken with permission from A Stevens and J Lowe. Human Histology, 2nd edition. Mosby, 1997

Fig 5.9 adapted with permission from C Haslett (editor). Davidson's Principles and Practice of Medicine, 18th edition. Churchill Livingston, 1999

Figs 5.19 reproduced with permission from M Makris and M Greaves. Blood in Systemic Disease. Mosby, 1997

Fig 6.14 adapted with permission from T Gordon-Smith and J Marsh. Medicine (Haematology Part 1). The Medicine Publishing Company, 2000

Figs 7.5, 7.6, 7.7, 7.8, 7.9, 7.10, 7.11, 7.12, 7.13, 7.14, 7.15, 7.16, 7.18 and 7.20 reproduced with permission form A V Hoffbrand and J Petit. Clinical Haematology 2nd edition. W B Saunders, 1994

Figs 8.1 and 8.4 adapted with permission from A V Hoffbrand, J Petit and P Moss. Essential Haematology, 4th edition. Blackwell Science, 2001

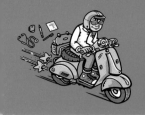

Dedication

To my girlfriend Mel and my father for their help, advice and support; to all my family and, in particular, to my mother who is always in my thoughts.

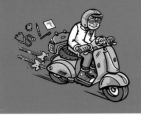

Contents

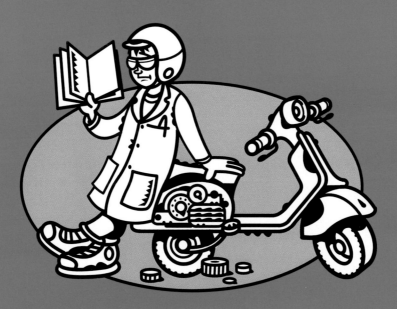

IMMUNOLOGY

1. Principles of Immunity

An overview of immunity

The human immune system has evolved over millions of years to protect against various challenges. The body is constantly exposed to infectious agents, including viruses, bacteria, protozoa, worms and other parasites. The human immune response must be varied because different organisms behave very differently and many pathogenic organisms have evolved mechanisms to survive the actions of the immune response.

The immune system can act rapidly but with little specificity. This initial immune response is known as the innate immune system. The innate immune system (see p. 8) consists of natural mechanical and chemical barriers to infection, cells and secreted proteins.

A more specific response, the adaptive immune system, takes a few days to be activated. The adaptive response is able to remember previously encountered pathogens and produce a larger and more rapid response if exposed to the same pathogen again. The innate components are thought to have a more ancient evolutionary origin than the adaptive components. A summary of the components of the innate and adaptive immune systems is given in Fig. 1.1.

Location of infection

To understand how the immune system functions it is important to look at the challenges it has to combat. The responses to intracellular and extracellular pathogens will be different. The size of the organism will also affect the immune response. Small organisms such as viruses can be phagocytosed by macrophages and neutrophils, whereas multicellular worms are too large to be taken up by immune cells.

Common pathogenic organisms and the immune response in different compartments of the body are shown in Fig. 1.2.

Defence against entry into the body

Physical and mechanical mechanisms provide the first line of defence against pathogenic infection (see p. 8). These are non-specific (innate) mechanisms. The innate immune system also employs chemicals to destroy or inactivate microorganisms and uses non-pathogenic microorganisms (normal flora) to inhibit colonization. Failure of these mechanisms can be due to host or factors associated with the pathogen (Fig. 1.3).

The pathogens

Once a pathogen has gained access to the body, a number of mechanisms are employed to combat infection. To understand which mechanisms are effective, it is necessary to look at the challenges particular pathogens provide.

Viruses

Viruses are small packages of genetic material. They are obligate intracellular parasites and must infect cells, where they use host machinery to replicate. Following viral replication, budding from the cell surface and release of new viral particles often causes the cell to lyse. Virus can be transported in the blood as free particles or spread directly from cell to cell.

Mechanisms by which the immune system targets viruses include:

- Inactivation of free virus by antibody
- Lysing of infected cells by CD8$^+$ T cells and natural killer (NK) cells
- Inhibition of viral replication in neighbouring cells by interferons.

The immune response against viruses is covered in more detail on page 39.

Bacteria

Bacteria are prokaryotic organisms. Their cell membrane is surrounded by a peptidoglycan cell wall; many bacteria also have a capsule of large branched polysaccharides. The cell wall and capsule protect the bacterium from phagocytosis. Bacterial infection is normally extracellular, however, some bacteria infect intracellularly.

Mechanisms by which the immune system targets extracellular bacteria include:

- Destruction of the cell wall and therefore lysis by complement and lysozyme
- Antipili antibodies prevent attachment
- Phagocytosis.

Components of the innate and adaptive immune systems		
	Innate system	Adaptive system
Cellular components	Monocytes/macrophages Neutrophils Eosinophils Basophils Mast cells Natural killer cells	B cells/Plasma cells T cells
Secreted components	Complement Cytokines Lysozyme Acute phase proteins Interferons	Antibody Cytokines

Fig. 1.1 Components of the innate and adaptive immune systems.

Site of infection				
	Extracellular		Intracellular	
	Interstitial spaces, blood, lymph	Epithelial surfaces	Cytoplasmic	Vesicular
Organisms	Transport of: Viruses Bacteria Protozoa Fungi Worms	Worms Most bacteria, e.g. *Neisseria gonorrhoeae,* *Streptococcus pneumoniae,* *Vibrio cholerae, Escherichia* *coli, Helicobacter pylori* Yeasts, e.g. *Candida albicans*	All viruses Protozoa *Chlamydia* spp. *Rickettsia* spp. *Listeria* *monocytogenes*	*Mycobacterium* *Salmonella* *typhimurium,* *Leishmania* spp. *Listeria* spp. *Trypanosoma* spp. *Legionella* *pneumophila,* *Cryptococcus* *neoformans,* *Yersinia pestis*
Host defence	Antibodies Complement Phagocytosis Neutralization	Antibodies (IgA) Antimicrobial peptides	Cytotoxic T cells NK cells	T cells and NK cells

Fig. 1.2 Infections at different body sites and mechanisms of host defence. IgA, immunoglobulin A; NK, natural killer.

Mechanisms by which the immune system targets intracellular bacteria include:
- Lysis of infected cells
- Prevention of spread (e.g. granuloma).

The immune response against bacteria is covered in more detail on page 41.

Protozoa
Protozoa are microscopic single-celled organisms. Immunity to protozoal infections is unlikely and disease is often chronic because:

- Infection is intracellular
- There is marked antigenic variation
- Infection is often immunosuppressive.

The immune response can target protozoa by:
- Preventing cellular penetration
- Cell-mediated lysis of infected cells
- Toxic actions of complement against protozoa.

The immune response against protozoa is covered in more detail on page 42.

Fig. 1.3 Failure of normal mechanisms to prevent infection.

Failure of mechanisms to prevent infection	
Failure of defence	**Pathogen (virulence) factors**
Dampness of the skin: can lead to damage and infection with fungi **Trauma:** if there is a break in the skin, microorganisms will infect the host more easily **Inoculation:** examples include intravenous drug abuse (*Staphylococcus aureus*), iatrogenic (following surgical procedures, etc.) or insect bites (e.g. mosquito bite allowing transmission of malaria) **Failure of clearance mechanisms in the lungs:** e.g. cystic fibrosis, results in recurrent lung infections **Antibiotic treatment:** can remove the normal flora	**Adhesion molecules:** e.g. bacterial pili, adhesions—enhance adherence **Motility and chemotaxis:** circumvents normal flushing mechanisms **Proteases:** digest mucus that prevents trapping **Active penetration:** larval stages of some helminths, e.g. hookworm, are able to penetrate intact skin

Worms

Worms are multicellular organisms, examples include roundworms (nematodes), flukes and tapeworms. They often have a complex lifecycle. Infection is normally by eggs, larvae or cysts that develop into worms within the host. Worms do not replicate within the host but will often be exposed to the immune system for a long time. To survive, they must be resistant to any immune response mounted against them.

The immune response targets worms by:
• Preventing implantation (by antibody and inflammation)
• Killing of certain worms (by eosinophils)
• Cell-mediated response to eggs.

As with protozoal infections, the immune response is rarely able to rid the host of infection and often causes most of the tissue damage resulting from infection.

Fungi

Fungi are simple organisms that lack chlorophyll, examples are moulds, yeasts and mushrooms. Fungi rarely infect humans, unless exposure is large or the patient is immunocompromised. Because of this, fungi are often described as 'opportunists'. Most infection is superficial, and deep infection can be fatal. Fungi can exhibit features that protect them from the immune system: antiphagocytic capsules, resistance to digestion by macrophages and destruction of polymorphs.

The immune response targets fungi by:
• Preventing entry to the body
• Phagocytosis (neutrophils)
• Killing (natural killer cell and CD8[+] T cells).

Defences once the microorganism penetrates the body

Both the innate and adaptive immune systems are involved in the response to pathogens. The systems overlap in their actions and the immune response to pathogens should be considered as a whole. The components of the immune system are outlined below.

Serum proteins
Complement

The complement system (see p. 14) consists of about 20 serum proteins. Complement has several actions, including lysis of bacteria and fungi, inflammation and opsonization (i.e. making more 'attractive' for phagocytes) of infected cells, bacteria and fungi.

Cytokines

Cytokines (see p. 7) are involved in both the innate and adaptive responses to pathogens. They can cause proliferation or activation of immune cells, mediate inflammation and produce an antiviral state in uninfected cells (interferons).

Acute phase proteins

Acute phase proteins are an innate response to infection. The liver is stimulated by cytokines and other factors to produce high levels of proteins that reduce bacterial toxicity and/or limit damage. Acute phase proteins include:

- C-reactive protein (see p. 13)
- α_1-antitrypsin
- α_1-antichymotrypsin
- Fibrinogen.

Antibody

Antibody is part of the adaptive immune response and is produced against most organisms. It works via a variety of mechanisms (see p. 27). Antibody cannot act directly against a pathogen while it is intracellular, but it might bind to the surface of the infected cell and activate other components of the immune system against the pathogen. Different types of antibody work at different sites within the body, e.g. secretory immunoglobulin A (sIgA) is involved with defence of mucosal surfaces.

Cells

Phagocytes

One of the most important innate responses to infection is phagocytosis (see p. 10), the process by which macrophages and neutrophils engulf small extracellular particles, e.g. bacteria or antigen–antibody complexes, and digest them.

The process of phagocytosis is enhanced by opsonization. This is enabled by certain substances such as antibody, known as opsonins, which bind to antigen.

Cytotoxic cells

Intracellular pathogens are shielded from most of the actions of the immune system. To destroy these pathogens, NK and cytotoxic T cells cause infected cells and fungi to undergo apoptosis or cell lysis (see p. 11).

Mast cells and basophils

Mast cells and basophils (see p. 11) are able to release many inflammatory mediators.

Eosinophils

Eosinophils are primarily involved in the response to helminths. They can release toxic mediators against the worm surface, and phagocytose antigen–antibody complexes.

Lymphocytes and antigen-presenting cells

Cytotoxic T cells have already been mentioned. Along with helper T cells, B cells and antigen-presenting cells, they mount a specific, adaptive immune response. B cells become plasma cells and produce antibody, and T helper cells and antigen-presenting cells control the response.

The response to tumours

Tumours, a neoplastic proliferation of host cells, provide a difficult challenge for the immune system. Most of the cell-surface antigens on the tumour will be the same as those on normal host cells. Most tumour cells are weakly antigenic and occasionally regress spontaneously. They also tend to be immunosuppressive.

It is also important to remember that cells of the immune system can undergo neoplastic change (see p. 103). Targets for the immune system on tumour cells include:

- Viral antigens (these occur in virus-induced tumours)
- Embryonic antigens, e.g. carcinoembryonic antigen in colon cancer, and α-fetoprotein in liver cancers
- Glycosylated variants of normal cell proteins
- High concentrations of normal self proteins
- Absence of major histocompatibility complex (MHC) class I molecules.

Antibody has little in vivo effect in tumour suppression, although passive administration of monoclonal antibody specific for tumour-associated antigens is being tested. Cytokines, tumour necrosis factor-α (TNF-α) and interleukin-1 (IL-1), are also being used therapeutically. An overview of the response to tumours is shown in Fig 1.4.

Immunity

Immunity is a state of relative resistance to disease.

Fig. 1.4 The immune response to tumours. Both innate and adaptive immunity have been implicated in the response to tumours. Macrophages can inhibit tumour growth or cause cytotoxicity, probably through the release of tumour necrosis factor-α (TNF-α). Complement activation may also cause tumour cell lysis. Cytotoxic CD8⁺ T cells have been shown to lyse tumour cells in vitro. Many tumours evade T cell cytotoxicity by reducing major histocompatibility complex (MHC) class I expression. This exposes them to lysis by natural killer (NK) cells. T helper cells activate cytotoxic T cells, macrophages and NK cells. They also produce TNF-β, which inhibits tumour growth.

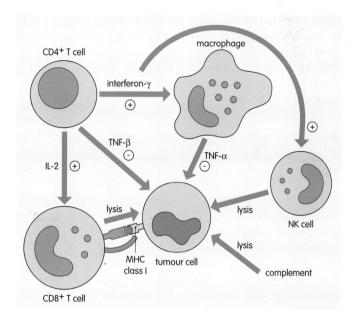

The innate and adaptive immune systems

Innate immunity provides a rapid response to a challenge. It is not antigen specific and does not change with repeated exposures.

Adaptive immunity is characterized by:

- **Specificity:** the ability to distinguish between different antigens
- **Memory:** the response is more rapid and occurs to a greater extent when exposed to an antigen for a second time (Fig 1.5).

Both the innate and adaptive immune systems comprise cellular and humoral components (see Fig. 1.1).

Cytokines

Cytokines are small, secreted proteins. They act locally, via specific cell-surface receptors, as part of both the innate and adaptive immune response. Cytokines have many effects, but in general they stimulate the immune response through:

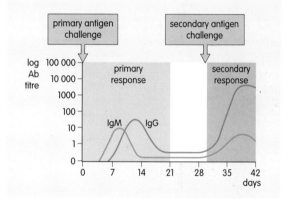

Fig. 1.5 Primary and secondary antibody (Ab) responses. IgM is the first antibody to be produced and is usually less specific than IgG that is produced subsequently. Following a second challenge with the same antigen, IgG is the primary antibody produced. It has a higher affinity for the antigen, is produced more rapidly, to greater titres and high levels persist for longer than in the primary response. Less IgM is produced during the secondary response.

An **antigen** is any molecule that can be recognized by the adaptive immune system. An **immunogen** is an antigen that evokes an immune response. Not all antigens are immunogens.

Epitopes are the small parts of the antigen recognized by the immune system. A single antigen can have more than one epitope, each of which is recognized by a different antibody or T cell receptor (TCR).

- Growth, activation and survival of various cells
- Increased production of surface molecules such as MHC.

Some important cytokines and their main actions are shown in Fig 1.6.

The innate immune system

Innate defences can be classified into three main groups:
1. Barriers to infection
2. Cells
3. Serum proteins and the complement system.

Barriers to infection
Physical and mechanical

Skin and mucosal membranes act as physical barriers to the entry of pathogens. Tight junctions between cells prevent the majority of pathogens from entering the body. The flushing actions of tears, saliva and urine protect epithelial surfaces from colonization. High oxygen tension in the lungs, and body temperature, can also inhibit microbial growth.

In the respiratory tract, mucus is secreted to trap microorganisms. They are then mechanically expelled by:
- Beating cilia (mucociliary escalator)
- Coughing
- Sneezing.

Important cytokines and their actions		
Cytokine	**Main sources**	**Main actions**
IL-1	Macrophages	Fever T-cell and macrophage activation
IL-2	T helper 1 cells	Growth of T cells Stimulates growth of B cells and NK cells
IL-3	T helper cells	Growth factor for progenitor haemopoietic cells
IL-4	T helper 2 cells	Activation and growth of B cells IgG1, IgE and MHC class II induction of B cells Growth and survival of T cells
IL-6	Macrophages	Lymphocyte activation Increased antibody production Fever, induces acute phase proteins
IL-8	Macrophages	Chemotactic factor for neutrophils Activates neutrophils
IL-10	T helper 2 cells Macrophages	Inhibits immune function
IL-12	Macrophages	Activates natural killer cells Causes CD4+ T cells to differentiate into T helper 1 cells
IFN	T helper 1 cells NK cells	Activation of macrophages and NK cells Produces antiviral state in neighbouring cells Increases expression of MHC class I and II molecules Inhibits T helper 2 cells
TNF-α	T helper cells Macrophages	Activates macrophages and induces nitric oxide production Proinflammatory Fever and shock
TNF-β	T helper 1 cells	Activates macrophages and neutrophils Induces nitric oxide production Kills T cells, fibroblasts and tumour cells

Fig. 1.6 Important cytokines and their actions. CTL, cytotoxic T lymphocyte; IL, interleukin; IFN, interferon; MHC, major histocompatibility complex; NK, natural killer; TNF, tumour necrosis factor.

8

Chemical
The growth of microorganisms is inhibited at acidic pH (e.g. in the stomach and vagina). Lactic acid and fatty acids in sebum (produced by sebaceous glands) maintain the skin pH between 3 and 5. Enzymes such as lysozyme (found in saliva, sweat and tears) and pepsin (present in the gut) destroy microorganisms.

Biological (normal flora)
A person's normal flora is formed when non-pathogenic bacteria colonize epithelial surfaces. Normal flora protects the host by:
- Competing with pathogenic bacteria for nutrients and attachment sites
- Production of antibacterial substances.

The use of antibiotics disrupts the normal flora and pathogenic bacteria are then more likely to cause disease.

Cells of innate immunity
Neutrophils
Neutrophils (for structure see p. 99, production p. 101) comprise 50–70% of circulating white cells. Neutrophils are the first cells to arrive at the site of inflammation and are the major constituent of pus. In response to tissue damage, neutrophils migrate from the bloodstream to the site of the insult (see Chapter 2). They are phagocytes and have an important role in engulfing and killing extracellular pathogens. The process of phagocytosis, and the mechanisms of killing are shown on page 10.

Mononuclear phagocyte system
Mononuclear phagocytes (for structure and production see p. 100) comprise the other major group of phagocytic cells. Monocytes account for 5–10% of the white cell count and circulate in the blood for approximately 8 hours before migrating into the tissues, where they differentiate into macrophages. Some macrophages become adapted for specific functions in particular tissues, e.g. Kupffer cells in the liver, glial cells in the brain. Monocytes also differentiate into osteoclasts and microglial cells.

In comparison to monocytes, macrophages:
- Are larger and longer-lived
- Have greater phagocytic ability
- Have a larger repertoire of lytic enzymes and secretory products.

Macrophages phagocytose and destroy their targets using similar mechanisms to neutrophils. The rate of phagocytosis can be greatly increased by opsonins such as IgG and C3b (neutrophils and macrophages have receptors for these molecules, which may be bound to the antigenic surface). Intracellular pathogens, e.g. *Mycobacterium*, can prove difficult for macrophages to kill. They are either resistant to destruction inside the phagosome or can enter the macrophage cytoplasm. For the immune system to act against these pathogens, T cell help is required.

In addition to phagocytosis, macrophages can secrete a number of compounds into the extracellular space, including cytokines (TNF and IL-1), complement components and hydrolytic enzymes. Macrophages are also able to process and present antigen in association with class II MHC molecules.

Macrophages express a wide array of surface molecules including:
- Fc-γRI–III (receptors for the Fc portion of IgG, types I–III) and complement receptors
- Receptors for bacterial constituents
- Cytokine receptors, e.g. TNF-α and IFN-γ
- MHC and B7 molecules (to activate the adaptive immune response).

Macrophages can be activated by:
- Cytokines such as IFN-γ
- Contact with complement or products of blood coagulation
- Direct contact with the target.

Following activation macrophages became more efficient phagocytes and have increased secretory and microbicidal activity. They also stimulate the adaptive immune system by expressing higher levels of MHC class II molecules.

In comparison to neutrophils, macrophages:
- Are longer-lived (they do not die after dealing with pathogens)
- Are larger (diameter 25–50µm), enabling phagocytosis of larger targets
- Move and phagocytose more slowly
- Exhibit a less pronounced respiratory burst
- Retain Golgi apparatus and rough endoplasmic reticulum and can therefore synthesize new proteins, including lysosomal enzymes and secretory products
- Secrete a variety of substances
- Can act as antigen-presenting cells (APCs).

Killing by phagocytes

The process of phagocytosis allows cells to engulf matter that needs to be destroyed. The cell can then digest the material in a controlled fashion before releasing the contents. The process of phagocytosis is shown in Fig. 1.7.

Microbial degradation within the phagolysosome occurs along two pathways; one requires oxygen, the other is oxygen independent.

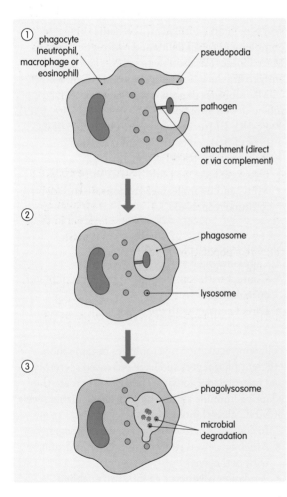

Fig. 1.7 Phagocytosis. Phagocytes sense an organism and bind it via non-specific receptors or via complement or antibody. Pseudopodia extend from the surface of the cell to surround the pathogen (1). The pseudopodia fuse around the organism, producing a vesicle known as a phagosome (2). Lysosomes fuse with the phagosome to form phagolysosomes (3). Chemicals within the lysosome, and other granules that fuse with the phagolysosome, lead to degradation of the organism. The microbial products are then released.

Oxygen-independent degradation

Neutrophil granules contain several antimicrobial agents including:

- Lysozyme (splits peptidoglycan)
- Lactoferrin and reactive nitrogen intermediates (which complex with, and deprive pathogens of, iron)
- Proteolytic enzymes (degrade dead microbes)
- Defensins, cathepsin G and cationic proteins (damage microbial membranes).

Oxygen-dependent degradation

A respiratory burst, increased oxygen consumption, accompanies oxygen-dependent degradation. Granule oxidases, along with NADPH and NADPH oxidase, reduce molecular oxygen to superoxide radicals ($O_2^{\bullet-}$), a reactive oxygen species. The following reactions also occur producing other reactive species:

$$2O_2^{\bullet-} + 2H^+ \rightarrow H_2O_2 + O_2$$

$$O_2^{\bullet-} + H_2O_2 \rightarrow OH^{\bullet} + OH^- + O_2$$

$$H_2O_2 + Cl^- \rightarrow OCl^- + H_2O$$
(catalysed by myeloperoxidase)

$$OCl^- + amine \rightarrow chloramines$$

Hypochlorus acid (HOCl) and chloramines are longer-lived than the other oxidizing agents and are probably the most important target killing compounds in vivo. If a target cannot be easily phagocytosed, there may be extracellular release of granule contents, causing tissue damage.

Natural killer (NK) cells

NK cells are non-T, non-B cells of lymphoid lineage. They are also known as large granular lymphocytes and comprise 5–10% of circulating lymphocytes. NK cells are primarily involved in killing tumours and cells infected with intracellular pathogen, primarily viruses, *Leishmania* and *Listeria monocytogenes*. NK cells are non-specifically activated by mitogens and the interferons, IL-2 and IL-12. NK cells are known as lymphokine-activated killer cells, because activation by IL-2, a lymphokine (produced by lymphoid cells), results in increased 'killing' ability.

Natural killer cells utilize cell-surface receptors to identify virally modified or cancerous cells. One set of receptors activates NK cells, initiating killing, others inhibit the cells:

- Activating receptors include calcium-binding C-lectins, which recognize certain cell-surface carbohydrates. Because these carbohydrates are present on the surface of normal host cells, a system of inhibitory receptors acts to prevent killing

- Killer inhibitor receptors (KIRs), members of the immunoglobulin gene superfamily, are specific for class I MHC molecules. Human natural killer cells also express an inhibitory receptor (a heterodimer CD94:NKG2) that detects non-classical class I molecules.

Virally infected cells often express reduced levels of MHC class I or, along with some tumour cells, altered class I MHC molecules. A reduction in MHC class I molecules avoids killing by cytotoxic CD8+ T cells, but make the cells susceptible to lysis by NK cells.

NK cells can also destroy antibody-coated target cells irrespective of the presence of MHC molecules, a process known as antibody-dependent cell-mediated cytotoxicity. This occurs because killing is initiated by cross-linking of receptors for the Fc portion of IgG1 and IgG3.

NK cells are not clonally restricted, have no memory and are not very specific in their action. They induce apoptosis in target cells (Fig. 1.8) by:

- Ligation of Fas or TNF receptors on the target cells (NK cells produce TNF and exhibit FasL). This initiates a sequence of caspase recruitment and activation, resulting in apoptosis
- Degranulation by NK cells, which releases perforins and granzymes. Perforin molecules

insert into and polymerize within the target cell membrane. This forms a pore through which granzymes can pass. Granzyme B then initiates apoptosis from within the target cell cytoplasm.

Eosinophils

Eosinophils (for structure see p. 100) comprise 1–3% of circulating white cells and are found principally in tissues. They are derived from the colony-forming unit for granulocytes, erythrocytes, monocytes and megakaryocytes (CFU-GEMM) haematopoietic precursor and their maturation is similar to that of the neutrophil (see p. 102). They are important in the defence against parasites and cause damage by extracellular degranulation. Their granules contain major basic protein, cationic protein, peroxidase and perforin-like molecules. Some of the products are anti-inflammatory and can inactivate mast cell products.

Basophils and mast cells

Basophils and mast cells (for structure see p. 101) have similar functions but are found in different locations; basophils comprise <1% of circulating white cells, whereas mast cells are resident in the tissues. This has led to the theory that mast cells are a population of differentiated basophils.

High concentrations of mast cells are found close to blood vessels in connective tissue, skin and mucosal membranes. The two types of mast cell,

Fig. 1.8 Mechanism of killing by natural killer (NK) cells (1). Activation of NK cells in the absence of an inhibitory signal results in degranulation (2). Perforins form a pore in the target cell allowing entry of granzymes (3). TNF produced by NK cells acts on target's cell receptors (4). FasL interacts with target cell Fas (5). Intracellular signalling from Fas, TNF receptors and granzymes results in apoptosis (6).

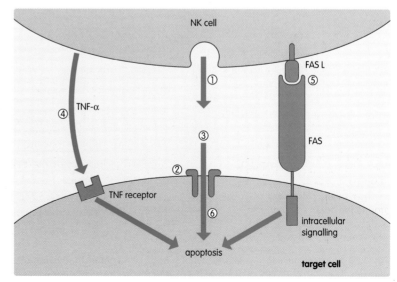

mucosal and connective tissue, differ in their tissue distribution, protease content and secretory profiles.

Mast cells function by discharging their granule contents. Degranulation is triggered by cross-linking of high-affinity receptors for the Fc portion of IgE (Fig. 1.9). Cross-linkage results in an influx of calcium ions into the cell, which induces release of pharmacologically active mediators from granules (Fig. 1.10). This is important in allergic responses (type I hypersensitivity reactions, see p. 43).

Soluble proteins
The soluble proteins that contribute to innate immunity (Fig. 1.11) can be divided into antimicrobial serum agents and proteins produced by cells of the immune system.

Acute phase proteins
The acute phase response is a systemic reaction to infection or tissue injury, e.g. inflammation, necrosis

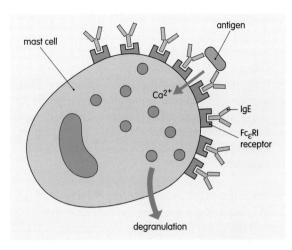

Fig. 1.9 Activation of mast cells by immunoglobulin E (IgE). IgE, produced by plasma cells, binds via its Fc domain to receptors on the mast cell surface. Cross-linking of these receptors by an antigen causes an influx of calcium ions into the cell. Calcium ions cause a rapid degranulation of inflammatory mediators from the mast cell.

	Mast cell granule contents	
Mediator		**Action**
Primary	Histamine	Increased capillary permeability, vasodilation, smooth muscle contraction
	Serotonin	Increased capillary permeability, vasodilation, smooth muscle contraction, platelet aggregation
	Heparin	Anticoagulation (see p. 122), modulates tryptase
	Proteases — Tryptase	Activates complement (C3)
	Proteases — Chymase	Increased mucus secretion
	Eosinophil chemotactic factor	Chemotactic (cells move towards site of production) for eosinophils
	Neutrophil chemotactic factor	Chemotactic for neutrophils
	Acid hydrolases	Degradation of extracellular matrix
	Platelet-activating factor	Platelet aggregation and activation, increased capillary permeability, vasodilation, chemotactic for leucocytes, neutrophil activation
Secondary	Leukotrienes (C_4, D_4, B_4)	Vasodilation, smooth muscle contraction, mucus secretion, chemotactic for neutrophils
	Prostaglandins (D_2)	Vasodilation, smooth muscle contraction, chemotactic for neutrophils, potentiation of other mediators
	Bradykinin	Increased capillary permeability, vasodilation, smooth muscle contraction, stimulation of pain nerve endings
	Cytokines	Various

Fig. 1.10 Mast cell mediators and their actions. Mast cells contain many preformed (primary) mediators that are stored in granules. They can also synthesize new (secondary) mediators when they are activated.

Soluble protein contributing to innate immunity		
	Protein	Notes
Secreted agents	Lysozyme	Bactericidal enzyme in mucus, saliva, tears, sweat and breast milk Cleaves peptidoglycan in the cell wall
Innate antimicrobial serum agents	Lactoferrin	Iron-binding protein that competes with microorganisms for iron, an essential metabolite
	Complement	Group of ~20 proenzymes Activation leads to an enzyme cascade, the products of which enhance phagocytosis and mediate cell lysis Alternative pathway can be activated by non-specific mechanism
	Mannan-binding lectin	Activates the complement system
	C-reactive protein	Acute phase protein, produced by the liver Serum concentration rises > 100-fold in tissue-damaging infections Binds C-polysaccharide cell wall component of bacteria and fungi Activates complement via classical pathway Opsonizes for phagocytosis
Proteins produced by cells of the innate system	Interferon-α Interferon-β	Produced by virally infected cells Induces a state of viral resistance in neighbouring cells by: • Inducing genes that will destroy viral DNA • Inducing MHC class I expression
	Interferon-γ	Mainly produced by activated NK cells Activates NK cells and macrophages

Fig. 1.11 The soluble proteins of innate immunity. MHC, major histocompatibility complex; NK, natural killer.

or malignancy. It is characterized by altered concentrations of a number of plasma proteins, acute phase proteins (APPs), which are produced by the liver. These include:
• C-reactive protein
• Serum amyloid A
• Complement components
• Fibrinogen
• α_1-Antitrypsin
• Caeruloplasmin
• Haptoglobulin.

The change in plasma concentration is accompanied by fever, leucocytosis, thrombocytosis and catabolism of muscle proteins. Synthesis of APPs is enhanced by cytokines secreted by macrophages and endothelial cells. The two main APPs are C-reactive protein (CRP) and serum amyloid A (SAA).

The extent of the rise in the plasma concentration of different APPs varies:
• Increased 50% above normal levels: caeruloplasmin
• Increased several fold above normal levels: α_1-glycoprotein, α_1-proteinase inhibitor, haptoglobulin, fibrinogen
• 100–1000-fold increase: CRP, SAA.

The concentration of other plasma proteins, most notably albumin and transferrin, falls.

C-reactive protein
Levels of CRP rise within hours of tissue injury or infection. The actions of CRP are outlined in Fig. 1.11. CRP elevation can be slight (e.g. cerebrovascular accident), moderate (e.g. myocardial infarction) or marked (e.g. bacterial infections).

Serum amyloid A
SAA levels rise within hours of tissue injury or infection. It may function as an opsonin. Persistent elevation of SAA can lead to its deposition in tissues in amyloidosis (see p. 111).

Erythrocyte sedimentation rate
The erythrocyte sedimentation rate (ESR) is an index of the acute phase response. It is especially

representative of the concentration of fibrinogen and α-globulins. Elevated fibrinogen levels cause red cells to form stacks (rouleaux), which sediment more rapidly than individual blood cells.

The complement system

The complement system consists of over 20 serum glycoproteins, synthesized principally by hepatocytes. The complement system is important for the recruitment of inflammatory cells, and the killing or opsonization of pathogens.

Many of the complement components circulate in the serum as proenzymes (functionally inactive enzymes) that require proteolytic cleavage for activation. The larger fragment binds to the surface of the substrate and the smaller one diffuses away. Once a component is activated, it catalyses the next step of the pathway. Components remain in the activated state for only a short time.

There are three pathways of complement activation—classical, lectin and alternative pathways—that terminate in a common final pathway. An overview of the complement system is given in Fig. 1.12.

The classical pathway

Antibodies (particularly IgG and IgM), bound to antigen, can activate the classical pathway via their CH2 or CH3 domains. C1 (a complex of one C1q and two C1s and C1r molecules) binds to immunoglobulin via the C1q component. This results in:

- Activation of C1r and C1s
- C1s activates C4, which then binds C2
- C2 is then activated by C1s
- Formation of C3 convertase (the C4b/C2a complex).

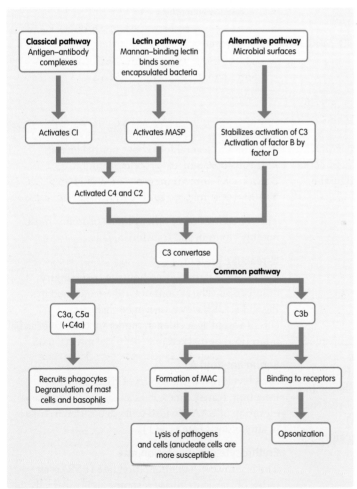

Fig. 1.12 Overview of the complement system. Cell lysis by complement is due to formation of the membrane attack complex (MAC). This is formed when C5b, C6, C7, C8 and C9 bind together to form a 10-nm pore in the cell surface. MASP, Mannan-binding lectin associated serine protease.

The lectin pathway

Mannan-binding lectin (MBL), which is normally found in serum, binds to MBL-associated serine proteases (MASP). This complex bears structural homology to the C1 complex. When MBL binds to carbohydrate on the surface of bacteria, MASP is activated. MASP then acts on C4 and C2 to generate the C3 convertase of the classical pathway.

The alternative pathway

C3 contains a labile thioester bond that is susceptible to spontaneous hydrolysis. C3b, generated in this way, is deposited on host and microbial surfaces. Certain features of microbial surfaces allow persistence of C3b:

- Lack of inactivatory regulatory molecules (present on eukaryotic cell membranes)
- On microbial surfaces, C3b tends to bind factor B rather than factor H (an inhibitory molecule).

Activation of factor B by factor D results in the formation of C3bBb, which is a C3 convertase.

The common terminal pathway

C5 convertase is formed from C3 convertase and C3b. Because C3 convertase is able to produce large quantities of C3b, it acts as a major amplification step in the complement pathway. Cleavage of C5 produces activated C5b, which sequentially binds C6, C7 and C8. C5b67 inserts into the cell membrane and C8 binds to this membrane-bound complex. Between 10 and 16 molecules of C9, a perforin-like molecule, bind to the C5b678 complex to create an ion-permeable pore. The C5b6789 complex, which is also called the membrane attack complex (MAC), results in osmotic lysis of the cell.

Functions of complement

The products of the complement pathway play an important role in both adaptive and innate immunity (Fig. 1.13).

Inhibitors of complement

Inhibitors of the complement pathway are important in regulating its activity and preventing complement-mediated damage of healthy cells. Factors that inhibit complement include:

- Membrane cofactor protein, complement receptor type 1, C4b-binding protein and factor H: these prevent assembly of C3 convertase
- Decay accelerating factor: this accelerates decay of C3 convertase
- C1 inhibitor: inhibits C1
- Factor I and membrane cofactor protein: cleave C3b an C4b
- CD59 (protectin): prevents the formation of membrane attack complex (MAC).

Recognition molecules

The immunoglobulin domain

B and T cell surface receptors are members of the immunoglobulin gene superfamily. Genes in this

Fig. 1.13 Functions of complement. MAC, membrane attack complex.

Functions of complement	
Function	Notes
Cell lysis	Insertion of MAC causes lysis of Gram-negative bacteria. Nucleated cells are more resistant to lysis because they endocytose MAC
Inflammation	C3a, C4a, C5a cause degranulation of mast cells and basophils C3a and C5a are chemotactic for neutrophils
Opsonization	Phagocytes have C3b receptors, which means that they are able to phagocytose antigen coated in C3b
Solubilization and clearance of immune complexes	Complement prevents immune complex precipitation and solubilizes complexes that have already been precipitated. Complexes coated in C3b bind to CR1 on red blood cells. The complexes are then removed in the spleen

family code for proteins composed of motifs called immunoglobulin domains. Members of this gene family include:

- Immunoglobulin (B cell receptor)
- T cell receptor
- MHC molecules
- T cell accessory molecules such as CD4
- Certain adhesion molecules, e.g. ICAM-1, ICAM-2 and VCAM-1
- Poly-Ig receptor
- Ig-α/Ig-β heterodimer.

Each domain is approximately 110 amino acids in length. The polypeptide chain in each domain is folded into seven or eight antiparallel beta strands. The strands are arranged to form two opposing sheets, linked by a disulphide bond and hydrophobic interactions. This compact structure is called the immunoglobulin fold.

Structure of B and T cell surface antigen receptors
Structure of immunoglobulin

The B cell surface receptor is a membrane-bound immunoglobulin (mIg) molecule. mIg recognizes the conformational structure (shape) of antigenic epitopes. Ig is composed of two light and two heavy chains. In the B cell receptor (Fig. 1.14), mIg associates with two Ig-α/Ig-β dimers (members of the immunoglobulin gene superfamily). Signal transduction through the mIg is thought to be mediated by the Ig-α/Ig-β heterodimers.

Ig is also secreted by plasma cells (see p. 23). The extracellular portion of mIg is identical in structure to secretory Ig. mIg differs from secreted Ig (sIg) because it has transmembrane and cytoplasmic portions that anchor it to the membrane. Different Ig classes can be expressed on the same B cell and may indicate the stage of development of the B cell, e.g. a mature, but antigenically unchallenged, B cell expresses both mIgM and mIgD. The antigenic specificity of all of the mIg molecules expressed on any given B cell is the same.

The T cell surface antigen receptor

Antigen recognition by T cells differs from antigen recognition by B cells:

- T cells recognize antigen only when it is associated with a molecule of the MHC
- T cells recognize peptide fragments of an antigen in association with MHC molecules, its not in original conformation. Therefore, antigen must be processed before it is presented to the T cell.

The T cell surface antigen receptor consists of the T cell receptor (TCR) associated with CD3. The TCR is a heterodimer, comprising α- and β-chains, or γ- and δ-chains. Approximately 95% of T cells express $\alpha\beta$-receptors. T cells expressing $\gamma\delta$-receptors are found particularly in epithelial tissues. The TCR is structurally similar to the immunoglobulin Fab region (see p. 24). Each chain comprises two immunoglobulin domains, one variable and one constant, linked by a disulphide bond. As in the variable domains of immunoglobulin, three variable regions on each chain combine to form the antigen-binding site.

CD3 is made up of three polypeptide dimers, consisting of four or five different peptide chains. The dimers are $\gamma\epsilon$, $\delta\epsilon$ and $\zeta\zeta$ (found in 90% of CD3 molecules) or $\zeta\eta$. The γ-, δ- and ϵ-chains are members of the Ig gene superfamily. The TCR recognizes and binds antigen, and CD3, functionally analogous to the Ig-α/Ig-β heterodimer in B cells, is involved in signal transduction (Fig. 1.15).

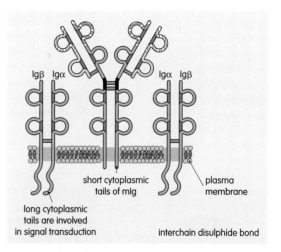

Fig. 1.14 Structure of the B cell surface receptor. Membrane-bound immunoglobulin is non-signalling. It associates with two Ig-α/Ig-β heterodimers (members of the immunoglobulin gene superfamily), which have long cytoplasmic domains capable of transducing a signal.

Fig. 1.15 Structure of the T cell surface antigen receptor. Negative charges on the transmembrane portion of CD3 components interact with positive charges on the T cell receptor (TCR). This maintains the complex. Antigen is detected by the TCR, but the signal is transduced by CD3.

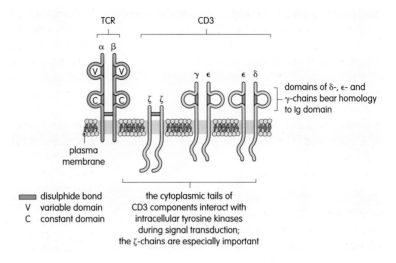

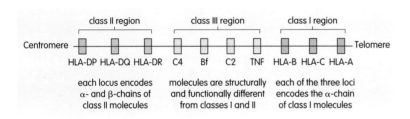

Fig. 1.16 Genetic organization of the human leucocyte antigen (HLA) complex. Only the classical genes are shown. The HLA complex is located in a 3–4 megabase sequence on the short arm of chromosome 6.

The major histocompatibility complex (MHC)

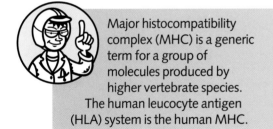

Major histocompatibility complex (MHC) is a generic term for a group of molecules produced by higher vertebrate species. The human leucocyte antigen (HLA) system is the human MHC.

The MHC is a cluster of tightly linked genes, found on the short arm of chromosome 6. Gene products of the MHC are involved in peptide binding, processing and presentation. Several complement proteins (C4, C2 and factor B), cytokines (TNF-α), transcription factors and enzymes are also encoded within the MHC. MHC molecules allow the immune system to detect self from non-self and to detect the presence of pathogens. T cells recognize antigen in the context of MHC molecules.

The MHC genes

A complete set of MHC alleles inherited from one parent is referred to as a haplotype.

MHC genes exhibit a high degree of polymorphism, i.e. they exhibit considerable diversity (there are more than 100 identified alleles for human leucocyte antigen B (HLA-B)). This means that most individuals will be heterozygous at most MHC loci and that any two randomly selected individuals are very unlikely to have identical HLA alleles. Diversity of the MHC increases the chance that a person will be able to mount an adaptive response against a pathogen. The genetic loci are tightly linked, so that a set is inherited from each parent. The genes are divided into three regions, each region encoding one of the three classes of the MHC; class I, class II and class III (Fig. 1.16). The MHC alleles exhibit codominance, which means that both alleles are expressed.

Structure and function of the MHC

Class I and class II MHC molecules are glycoproteins expressed on the cell surface and consist of cytoplasmic, transmembrane and extracellular portions (Fig 1.17). Both class I and class II molecules exhibit broad specificity in their binding of peptide. The polymorphism of the MHC is largely concentrated in the peptide binding cleft. A summary of the differences between class I and II MHC molecules is shown in Fig. 1.18.

MHC restriction

T cells are only able to recognize antigen in the context of self-MHC molecules (self-MHC

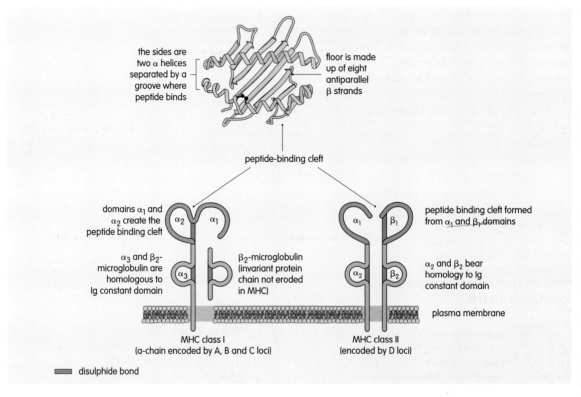

the sides are two α helices separated by a groove where peptide binds

floor is made up of eight antiparallel β strands

peptide-binding cleft

domains α₁ and α₂ create the peptide binding cleft

α₃ and β₂-microglobulin are homologous to Ig constant domain

β₂-microglobulin (invariant protein chain not eroded in MHC)

peptide binding cleft formed from α₁ and β₁ domains

α₂ and β₂ bear homology to Ig constant domain

plasma membrane

MHC class I (a-chain encoded by A, B and C loci)

MHC class II (encoded by D loci)

disulphide bond

Fig. 1.17 Structure of class I and class II major histocompatibility molecules (MHC). The peptide binding cleft of a class I molecule is also shown as seen from above.

Differences between class I and class II major histocompatibility molecules		
	Class I	**Class II**
Size of bound peptide	8–9 amino acids	13–18 amino acids (binding cleft more open)
Peptide from	Cytosolic antigen	Intravesicular or extracellular antigen
Expressed by	All nucleated cells, especially T cells, B cells, macrophages, other antigen-presenting cells, neutrophils	B cells, macrophages, other antigen-presenting cells, epithelial cells of the thymus, activated T cells
Recognized by	CD8⁺ T cells	CD4⁺ T cells

Fig. 1.18 Differences between class I and class II major histocompatibility molecules.

restriction). CD8$^+$ T cells recognize antigen only in association with class I MHC molecules (class I MHC restricted). CD4$^+$ T cells recognize antigen only in association with class II MHC molecules (class II MHC restricted).

Antigen processing and presentation

MHC molecules do not present whole antigen. The antigen is degraded into peptide fragments before binding can occur. There are different pathways of antigen processing for class I and class II MHC. The pathways are summarized in Fig. 1.19.

Professional antigen-presenting cells (APCs) process and present antigen to CD4$^+$ T cells in association with class II molecules. These cells express high levels of class II MHC molecules. Professional APCs include:

- Dendritic cells, including Langerhans' cells
- Macrophages
- B cells.

Structure and function of CD4 and CD8

CD4 and CD8 are 'accessory' molecules that play an important role in the T cell–antigen interaction. CD4 and CD8 have two important functions:

- They bind MHC class II and class I molecules, respectively, thereby strengthening the T cell–antigen interaction
- They function as signal transducers.

The role of CD4 and CD8 in antigen–receptor binding is shown in Fig. 1.20.

Generation of antigen receptor diversity

Because of the diversity of antigen that the body encounters, antigen receptors must also be diverse. Diversity is primarily produced within the variable domains of immunoglobulin and the TCR.

Fig. 1.19 Routes of antigen processing. (1) Class I molecules present endogenous antigens. Cytosolic antigen is degraded by proteosomes and transported into the rough endoplasmic reticulum (ER), where peptides are loaded onto class I molecules. The MHC–peptide complex is transported via the Golgi apparatus to the cell surface. (2) Class II molecules present exogenous antigens that have been phago- or endocytosed into intracellular vesicles. The MHC molecule is transported from the rough ER to the vesicle by the invariant chain (Ii). It is displaced from the MHC molecule by processed antigen, which is then presented at the cell surface. MHC, major histocompability complex.

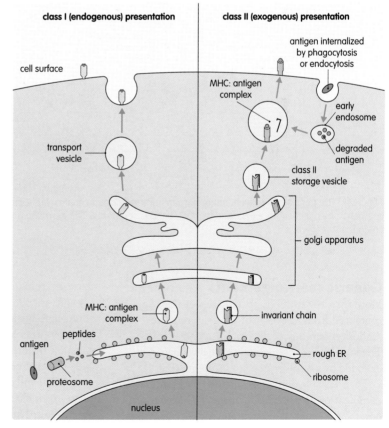

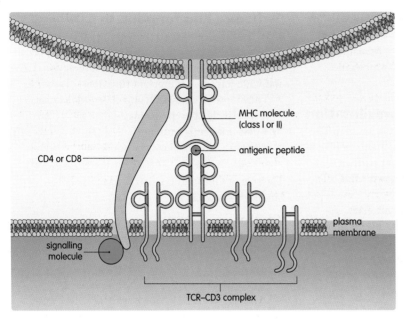

Fig. 1.20 The role of CD4 and CD8 in T cell receptor (TCR)–major histocompatibility complex (MHC) antigen interaction. CD4 or CD8 is closely associated with the TCR complex. They bind MHC in a restricted fashion (CD8 to class I only, CD4 to class II only). Binding is antigen independent and strengthens the bond between TCR and a complementary peptide–MHC complex. Molecules associated with CD4 or CD8 are then able to transduce a signal.

chain	Chromosome	Number of gene segments			
		V	D	J	C
κ light chain	2	~100	–	5	1
λ light chain	22	~100	–	6	6
heavy chain	14	75–250	30	6	9

Gene segments encoding immunoglobulin chains in humans

5′ ▪ ▪ / ▪ // ☐ ☐ ☐ ☐ ☐ ☐ 3′
 V_{κ1} V_{κ2} V_{κn} J_{κ1} J_{κ2} J_{κ3} J_{κ4} J_{κ5} C_{κ}

5′ ▪ ▪ / ▪ // ☐ ☐ / ☐ ☐ ☐ / ☐ ▪ ▪ ▪ ▪ ▪ ▪ ▪ ▪ ▪ 3′
 V_{H1} V_{H2} V_{Hn} D_1 D_2 D_n J_{H1} J_{H2} J_{H6} C_μ C_δ C_{γ3} C_{γ1} C_{α1} C_{γ2} C_{γ4} C_ε C_{α2}

Fig. 1.21 The gene segments encoding human immunoglobulin chains. Light chains are composed of V, J and C segments; heavy chains are encoded by V, D, J and C segments. The germline organization of the κ light chain and heavy chain is also shown.

Genetic rearrangements

More than 10^8 antibody specificities can be generated from just 0.1% of the genome. The random generation of diversity has a genetic basis. The κ and λ light chains and the heavy chain are encoded by a number of gene segments (Fig. 1.21).

Each variable domain is encoded by a random combination of one of each of the V, D (heavy chain only) and J exons. Following genetic rearrangement,

one exon remains which codes for an Ig domain. The C exons encode the constant regions. Heavy-chain C gene segments are clusters of exons, each of which encodes either a domain or hinge region of the constant region.

Following rearrangement, the clonal progeny of each B cell will produce Ig of a single specificity. Rearrangement is completed and functional Ig chains are produced before the B cell encounters antigen

(Figs. 1.22 and 1.23). The presence of multiple V, D (heavy chain only) and J gene segments, and the apparently random selection of these segments, generates considerable diversity, which can be calculated (Fig. 1.24).

A similar process occurs in T cells: α- and γ-chain variable domains have V and J segments; β- and δ-chain have V, D and J segments.

Allelic exclusion

This is the process whereby a B cell expresses only one set of heavy chain genes and only one set of light chain genes, thus ensuring that the antigenic specificity of the two halves of the Ig molecule is the same and that any B cell expresses immunoglobulin of only one specificity. Production of a functional heavy or light chain prevents rearrangement of the other sets of genes.

Junctional diversity

Several mechanisms are employed to create further diversity within the variable regions.

Junctional flexibility and N-nucleotide addition

When exons are spliced, there are slight variations in the position of segmental joining. In addition, up to 15 nucleotides can be added to the D–J and the V–DJ joints. This occurs only in heavy chains and is catalysed by terminal deoxynucleotidyl transferase.

Both junctional flexibility and N-nucleotide addition can disrupt the reading frame, leading to non-functional rearrangements. However, formation of productive rearrangements increases antibody diversity. The V–J, V–DJ and VD–J joints fall within the antigen-binding region of the variable domain. Therefore, diversity generated at these joints will impact on the antigen specificity of the Ig molecule.

Somatic hypermutation

During the course of a primary immune response, point mutations occur in the variable region exons of the Ig molecule. The resultant Ig molecules may have altered affinity for antigen. Those with higher affinities are positively selected because of clonal antigen drive. Antibodies produced later in the primary immune response, and in the secondary immune response, will therefore have an increased affinity for antigen (affinity maturation).

The TCR does not exhibit somatic hypermutation. This is probably because T cells do not recognize self-peptides, and only recognize self-MHC. Therefore diversity is generated only in

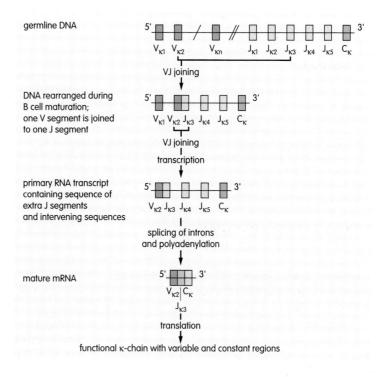

Fig. 1.22 Rearrangement of gene segments in the κ light chain. This process occurs during B-cell maturation and is not reversible.

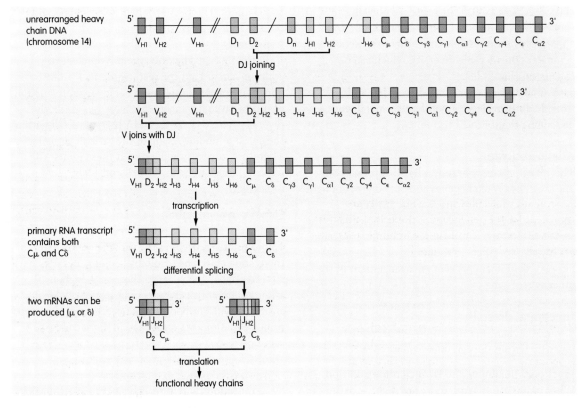

Fig. 1.23 Rearrangement of the heavy chain is similar to that of the light chain, although the join between D and J segments occurs first. In an unstimulated B cell, the heavy-chain mRNA that is transcribed contains both the Cμ and Cδ segments. The mRNA can be differentially spliced such that both IgM and IgD will be produced. They will both exhibit the same antigen binding specificity.

Calculation of antibody diversity			
Mechanism of diversity	**Number of combinations**		
	κ light chain	**λ light chain**	**Heavy chain**
Random joining of gene segments	$100 \times 5 = 500$	$100 \times 6 = 600$	$75 \times 30 \times 6 = 13\,500$
Random chain associations	$(500 + 600) \times 13\,500 = 1.5 \times 10^7$		

Fig. 1.24 Calculation of antibody diversity. Given the fact that light chain can associate with any heavy chain, and from the number of gene segments present in germline DNA, it is possible to calculate the number of different molecules that can be produced. The extent of the contribution of junctional flexibility, N-nucleotide addition and somatic hypermutation is not known but will be significant.

developing T cells, which can be deleted if they are either self reactive or non-functional.

Class switching
This is the process whereby a single B cell can produce different classes of Ig that have the same specificity. The mechanism is not well understood but involves 'switch sites'—DNA sequences located upstream from each heavy chain C gene segment (except C_δ). Possible mechanisms include:
• Differential splicing of the primary transcript (see Fig. 1.23)

- A looping out and deletion of intervening heavy chain C gene segments (and introns)
- Exchange of C gene segments between chromosomes.

This process underlies the class switch from IgM in the primary response, to IgG, IgA or IgE in the secondary response. Cytokines are important in controlling the switch.

The adaptive immune system

Recognition molecules and their diversity are important for the generation of a specific, adaptive immune response. The adaptive immune response can be humoral or cell-mediated.

Humoral immunity

B cells and antibody production

The humoral immune response is brought about by antibodies, which are particularly efficient at eliminating extracellular pathogens. Antigen can be cleared from the host by a variety of effector mechanisms, which are dependent on antibody class or isotype (see p. 27):
- Activation of complement, leading to lysis or opsonization of the microorganism
- Antibody-dependent cell-mediated cytotoxicity (ADCC)
- Neutralization of bacterial toxins and viruses
- Mucosal immunity (IgA-mediated).

Activated and differentiated B cells, known as plasma cells, produce antibodies. An overview of B cell activation is given in Fig. 1.25. B cells are activated within follicles found in secondary lymphoid structures, e.g. lymph nodes and spleen. B cells become activated only if they encounter specific antigen. During proliferation, variable regions of the immunoglobulin genes undergo somatic hypermutation (see p. 25). This process occurs in the germinal centre of the follicle. Follicular dendritic cells present antigen, to which the B cell clones with the highest affinity will bind. This causes the expression of bcl-2, which prevents B cells undergoing apoptosis. Therefore, the highest-affinity clones are positively selected. B cells that respond to soluble antigen or do not receive T cell help undergo apoptosis—negative selection of self-reactive and

non-reactive clones. An overview of clonal selection of B cells is given in Fig. 1.26.

T-cell-dependent and T-cell-independent antigens

The process shown in Fig. 1.25 illustrates the need for T cells in the activation of a humoral response. The antigens that trigger this process are therefore known as T-cell-dependent antigens. Not all antigens require T cells to produce an antibody response. T-cell-independent antigens, including many microbial constituents, are able to stimulate B cells directly or with the help of non-thymus-derived accessory cells.

Structure and function of antibody

The structure of immunoglobulin is shown in Fig. 1.27. Immunoglobulin molecules (using IgG as an example) are composed of two identical heavy and two identical light chains, linked by disulphide bridges. The light chains consist of one variable and three or four constant domains, depending on the class of antibody. Digestion of IgG with papain produces two types of fragment:
1. Two Fab fragments (bind antigen) consisting of the light chain and two domains of the heavy chain (denoted VH and CH1)
2. One Fc fragment (binds complement) consisting of the remainder of the heavy chain (CH2 and CH3).

The light chain
The light chain comprises two domains:
- The amino (N) terminal domain is variable and is the site of antigen binding
- The constant domain at the carboxy (C) terminal.

The constant region can be κ or λ, but both light chains within an Ig molecule will be the same; ~60% of human light chains are κ.

The heavy chain
The heavy chain has a variable domain attached to several constant domains. There are five classes of immunoglobulin (Ig) in humans, IgG, IgA, IgM, IgE and IgD. The heavy chain determines the immunoglobulin class. The heavy chain can be γ (IgG), α (IgA), μ (IgM), ε (IgE) or δ (IgD). IgG, IgA and IgD have three constant domains with a hinge region, IgM and IgE have four constant domains but no hinge region.

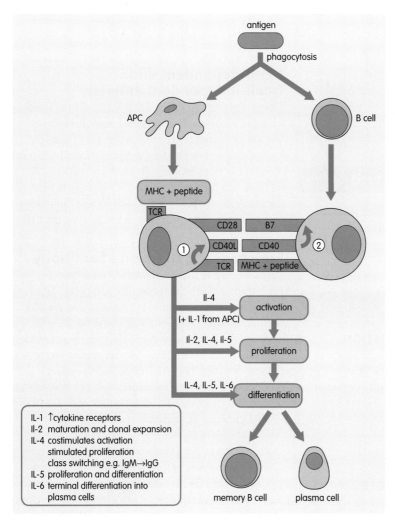

Fig. 1.25 Overview of the humoral immune response. Activated and differentiated B cells, known as plasma cells produce antibody. B cells are activated by antigen in a T-cell-independent or dependent fashion (only T-cell-dependent antigens are shown). T helper cells are primed by antigen-presenting cells (APCs), which present antigen in conjunction with MHC class II molecules. B cells are stimulated by antigen interacting with B cell receptors. Primed T helper cells interact with B cells that also express antigen–MHC complexes. This interaction induces a sequence of surface receptor binding and cytokine production that results in B-cell activation, proliferation and differentiation. (1) Binding of the T cell receptor (TCR) to MHC induces the T cell to produce CD40L, which binds to CD40 on the B cell, producing a major stimulatory signal. (2) CD28 on the T cell then interacts with B7 on the B cell (costimulatory signal). Cytokines are also involved, their actions are shown in the diagram.

The variable domain

Each variable domain exhibits three regions that are hypervariable. The hypervariable regions on both light and heavy chains are closely aligned in the immunoglobulin molecule. Together, they form the antigen-binding site and therefore determine the molecule's specificity. Because they must be complementary to the epitope they bind to, the hypervariable regions can be referred to as the complementarity-determining regions.

The hinge region

The hinge is a peptide sequence located between the first and second constant domains in the heavy chain. It allows the Fab regions to move against the Fc region from 0 to 90°. This allows greater interaction with epitopes. The hinge region is also the site of the interchain disulphide bonds.

Classes of antibody

Different classes and subclasses of antibody are known as **isotypes** or **allotypes**.

The **idiotype** of an antibody is how the unique features of the variable domains function as epitopes (**idiotopes**), which will bind a variety of **anti-idiotype** antibodies.

Haptens are small molecules that need to be bound to a large carrier molecule to be immunogenic.

Fig. 1.26 Clonal selection of B cells. During B cell activation, the antigen-binding region of the immunoglobulin gene undergoes hypermutation. Clonal selection ensures that cells that produce the best antibody are selected and that non-functional or self-reactive B cells are deleted. This process occurs within the germinal centres of lymphoid follicles.

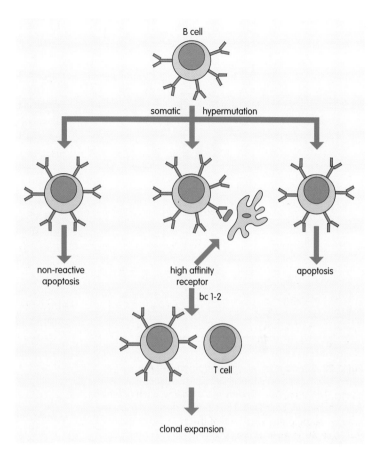

The different properties of the immunoglobulin classes are shown in Fig. 1.28. Different Ig classes and subclasses are specific to each species. IgG, IgE and IgD are monomeric, secreted IgA (sIgA) is usually present as a dimer, and secreted IgM as a pentamer. The sIgA molecule is made up of two IgA monomers, a J chain and a secretory piece. The IgA dimer (+J chain) is produced by submucosal plasma cells and enters the mucosal epithelial cell via receptor-mediated endocytosis, binding to the poly-Ig receptor. Having passed from the basal to the luminal surface of the epithelial cell, the IgA dimer is secreted across the mucosa, with part of the poly-Ig receptor (the secretory piece) still attached.

The functions of antibodies
The functions of Igs are shown in Fig. 1.29.

Lymphatic drainage and lymph nodes
Lymph nodes are secondary lymphoid organs. They provide a site for lymphocytes to interact with antigen and other cells of the immune system.

At the arterial end of capillaries, water and low-molecular-weight solutes leak out into tissue spaces, to create interstitial fluid. Most interstitial fluid returns to the venous circulation at the venous end of capillaries (due to pressure gradients). The remainder leaves the interstitial space via the lymphatic system. Once interstitial fluid has entered a lymphatic vessel it is known as lymph. Lymphatic vessels are present in almost all tissues and organs of the body.

Lymphatic circulation
The lymphatic system acts as a passive drainage system to return interstitial fluid to the systemic circulation; lymph is not pumped around the body. Lymph vessels therefore contain numerous valves to prevent backflow of lymph. Afferent lymph vessels carry lymph into lymph nodes. They empty into the subcapsular sinus and lymph percolates through the node. Each node is drained by only one efferent vessel.

Lymph returns to the circulation at lymphovenous junctions. These are located at the junction of the right subclavian vein and right internal jugular vein

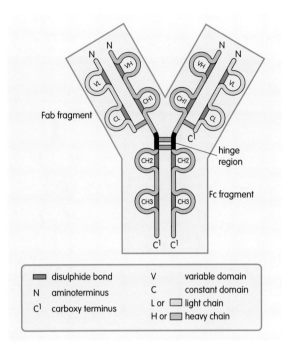

Fab fragment

hinge region

Fc fragment

disulphide bond	V	variable domain
N aminoterminus	C	constant domain
C¹ carboxy terminus	L or ▭ light chain
	H or ▭ heavy chain

Fig. 1.27 Structure of IgG. Immunoglobulins are composed from two identical light and two identical heavy chains. The chains are divided into domains, each of which is an immunoglobulin fold. The variable domains form the antigen-binding site. Digestion of the immunoglobulin molecule with papain produces an Fc portion (which binds complement) and two Fab portions (which bind antigen).

(which empties the right lymphatic duct) and at the junction of the left subclavian vein and left internal jugular vein (which empties the thoracic duct).

Lymph nodes

Lymph nodes act as filters, 'sampling' lymphatic fluid for bacteria, viruses and foreign particles. Antigen-presenting cells (APCs), loaded with antigen, also migrate through lymph nodes. They are present throughout the lymphatic system, often occurring at junctions of the lymphatic vessels. Lymph nodes frequently form chains, and may drain a specific organ or area of the body.

Lymph node structure

The structure of lymph nodes can be divided into three areas (Fig. 1.30):

1. **Cortex:** mainly B cells, initially organized as primary follicles. B cells sample antigen from

interstitial fluid that has been drained in the lymph and trapped on the surface of follicular dendritic cells. When stimulated by antigen, secondary follicles form, each containing a germinal centre that produces large numbers of plasma cells and memory B cells

2. **Paracortex:** T cells and dendritic cells (APCs expressing high levels of class II MHC molecules). Activation of T cells (by antigen presented by dendritic cells and B cells) and interaction with B cells is needed to produce antibodies

3. **Central medulla:** cellular cords that are populated with B and T lymphocytes, plasma cells and macrophages. The cords are located around medullary sinuses. The lymph drains into a terminal sinus, which eventually forms the efferent lymphatic vessel.

Lymph nodes act as sites for initiation of the adaptive immune response. Antigen is sampled, processed and presented by several professional APCs (macrophages and dendritic cells).

Lymphocyte recirculation

Lymphocytes move continuously between blood and lymph. Efferent lymph contains more lymphocytes than afferent lymph because:

- Antigenic challenge results in stimulation and proliferation of lymphocytes
- Lymphocytes enter the lymph node directly from blood.

Lymphocyte recirculation is essential for a normal immune response (Fig. 1.31). Approximately 1–2% of the lymphocytic pool recirculates each hour. This increases the chances of an antigenically committed lymphocyte encountering complimentary antigen.

Lymphocytes tend to recirculate to similar tissues. For example, an activated lymphocyte that has migrated from the skin to a local lymph node is most likely to migrate to another lymph node draining skin following transport in the blood. Similarly, lymphoctes activated in mucosal-associated lymphoid tissue (MALT) will return to MALT. This recirculation is governed by the expression of molecules on both the lymphocyte and surface endothelium. Areas of endothelium through which lymphocytes migrate are known as high endothelial venules (HEV). Lymphocytes activated in MALT express $\alpha_4\beta_7$ integrins that interact with MadCAM-1, an adhesion molecule only expressed on HEV in MALT tissue.

Properties of the five immunoglobulin classes					
	IgG	IgA	IgM	IgE	IgD
Physical properties					
Molecular weight (kDa)	150	300	900	190	150
Serum concentration (mg/mL)	13.5	3.5	1.5	0.0003	0.03
Number of subunits	1	2	5	1	1
Heavy chain	γ	α	μ	ε	δ
Subclasses	4	2	—	—	—
Biological activities					
Present in secretions	✗	✓	✓	✗	✗
Crosses placenta	✓	✗	✗	✗	✗
Complement fixation	✓	✓	✓✓✓	✗	✗
Binds phagocytic receptors	✓	✗	✓	✗	✗
Binds mast cell receptors	✗	✗	✗	✓	✗
Other features					
Main role	Main circulatory Ig for secondary immune response	Major Ig in secretions	Main Ig in primary immune response	Allergy and antiparasitic response	Expressed on naïve B cell; function not known

Fig. 1.28 Properties of the five immunoglobulin (Ig) classes.

Fig. 1.29 Summary of the functions of immunoglobulins. sIgA, secretory immunoglobulin A; NK, natural killer.

Functions of immunoglobulin	
Function	**Notes**
Opsonization	Phagocytic cells have antibody (Fc) receptors, thus antibody can facilitate phagocytosis of antigen
Agglutination	Antigen and antibody (IgG or IgM) clump together because immunoglobulin can bind more than one epitope simultaneously. IgM is more efficient because it has a high valency (10 antigen-binding sites)
Neutralization	Binding to pathogens or their toxins prevents their attachment to cells
Antibody-dependent cell-mediated cytotoxicity (ADCC)	The antibody–antigen complex can bind to cytotoxic cells (e.g. cytotoxic T cells, NK cells) via the Fc component of the antibody, thus targeting the antigen for destruction
Complement activation	IgG and IgM can activate the classical pathway; IgA can activate the alternative pathway
Mast cell degranulation	Cross-linkage of IgE bound to mast cells and basophils results in degranulation
Protection of the neonate	Transplacental passage of IgG and the secretion of sIgA in breast milk protect the newborn

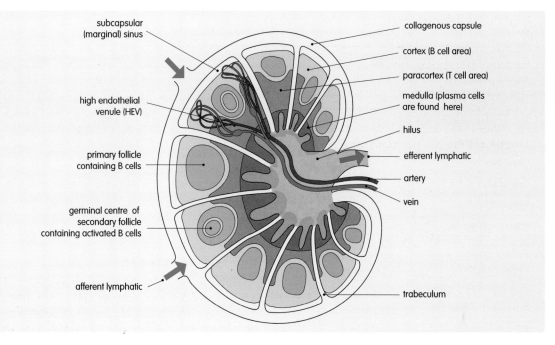

Fig. 1.30 Lymph node structure. A collagenous capsule through which several afferent lymphatic vessels pass surrounds lymph nodes. Lymph is deposited in the subcapsular sinuses and then drains through the cortex, paracortex and into the medulla where it drains into the efferent lymph. The blood supply to the lymph node consists of an artery and a vein through which lymphoid cells can pass. The lymph node provides a good environment for initiation of an adaptive immune response.

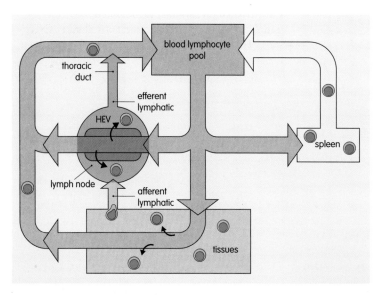

Fig. 1.31 Lymphocyte recirculation. Lymphocytes can enter lymph nodes via specialized high endothelial venules or in lymph. They leave the node in lymph that is returned to the systemic circulation via the right lymphatic duct or thoracic duct. HEV, high endothelial venule.

Lymphadenopathy

Lymph nodes can become enlarged (lymphadenopathy) for several reasons, including infection. Causes of lymphadenopathy can be seen on page 102.

Mucosal-associated lymphoid tissue (MALT)

MALT consists of unencapsulated subepithelial lymphoid tissue found in the gastrointestinal, respiratory and urogenital tracts (Fig. 1.32). It can be subdivided into:

- Organized lymphoid tissue, e.g. tonsils, appendix, Peyer's patches
- Diffuse lymphoid tissue located in the lamina propria of intestinal villi and lungs.

Organized lymphoid tissue
Respiratory tract
MALT tissue in the nose and bronchi includes the:
- Lingual, palatine and nasopharyngeal tonsils

- Adenoids
- Bronchial nodules.

The respiratory system is exposed to a large number of organisms every day, most of which are cleared by the mucociliary escalator. Microorganisms that are not removed are presented by dendritic cells in the bronchi and stimulate germinating centres.

Gastrointestinal tract
Peyer's patches are organized submucosal lymphoid follicles present throughout the large and small intestine, being particularly prominent in the lower ileum. The structure of a Peyer's patch is shown in Fig. 1.33.

Lymphocyte trafficking in MALT
Mucosal lymphocytes generally recirculate within the mucosal lymphoid system. This occurs through recognition between specific adhesion molecules on the surfaces of lymphocytes from Peyer's patches and corresponding ligands on the venular endothelium.

Cell-mediated immunity

Cell-mediated immunity is mediated by T lymphocytes, macrophages and natural killer (NK) cells. The cell-mediated immune system is involved in the elimination of:
- Intracellular pathogens and infected cells
- Tumour cells
- Foreign grafts.

The thymus plays an important role in cell-mediated immunity because it is the site of T-cell maturation.

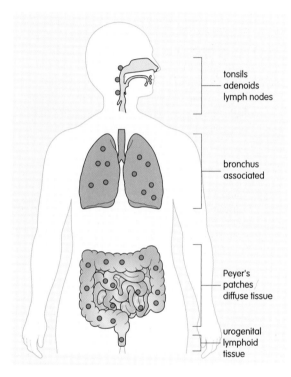

Fig. 1.32 Anatomical location of mucosal-associated lymphoid tissue (MALT). MALT is found in the nasal cavity, throat, respiratory tract, gastrointestinal tract and urogenital tract. Immune cells activated in MALT will home only to other mucosal sites.

Fig. 1.33 Structure of a Peyer's patch. Peyer's patches are found in the gastrointestinal tract. Microbes are transported across specialized epithelial M cells in pinocytotic vesicles into a dome-shaped area. Antigen-presenting cells then process and present antigen to T cells. Helper T cells can then activate B cells within the follicle.

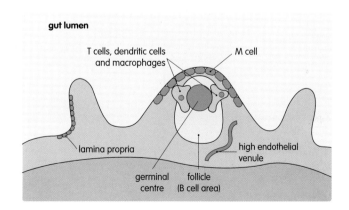

29

The thymus gland

The thymus is important for the production of T lymphocytes. T lymphocyte differentiation begins in the bone marrow (see. p. 69) before early precursor cells migrate to the thymus. In the thymus, immature T lymphocytes undergo random recombination of their T cell receptor genes. Some of the resulting T cell receptors will be specific for pathogens and others for normal self-antigens. The role of the thymus is to select T cells that will respond to pathogens but not self antigens.

The thymus is a gland with two lobes, located in the anterior part of the superior mediastinum; posterior to the sternum and anterior to the great vessels and upper part of the heart (Fig. 1.34). It can extend superiorly into the roof of the neck and inferiorly into the anterior mediastinum. It receives its blood supply from the inferior thyroid and internal thoracic arteries. Each lobe is surrounded by a capsule and divided into multiple lobules by fibrous septa known as trabeculae. Each lobule is divided into two regions (Fig. 1.35):

1. An outer cortex
2. An inner medulla.

Immature thymocytes (T cell progenitors) enter the thymus gland via the cortex, where they rapidly proliferate and rearrange their T cell receptor genes. T cells that recognize self antigen in the thymus are forced to undergo apoptosis—negative selection. T cells that are able to bind MHC to some extent will proliferate—positive selection. A much smaller and more mature group of thymocytes survives to enter the medulla. Thymocytes continue to mature in the

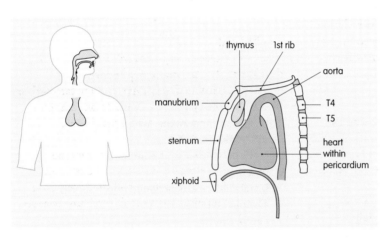

Fig. 1.34 Location of the thymus. The thymus is located in the superior mediastinum, behind the sternum, but above and in front of the heart. It can extend into the neck. After puberty the thymus reduces in size.

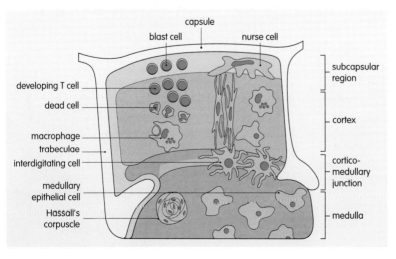

Fig. 1.35 Structure of a thymic lobule. The thymus is a bilobed gland, surrounded by a collagenous capsule, which is subdivided into lobules. Developing T cells (thymocytes) move from the subcapsular region to the medulla during maturation. Several different types of stromal cells support them. Many thymocytes undergo apoptosis (particularly in the cortex) and are phagocytosed by macrophages.

medulla and eventually leave the thymus, via postcapillary venules, as mature, antigen-specific, immunocompetent T cells. In total, only 1–5% of thymocytes in the thymus reach maturity, the remainder undergo programmed cell death (apoptosis).

Stromal cells of the thymus

The remainder of the thymic lobule is composed of a network of epithelial cells, known collectively as stromal cells. They interact with developing thymocytes and produce several hormones that are essential for their differentiation and maturation.

Embryological origin of the thymus

The human embryonic thymus develops from the third pharyngeal pouch during week 4 or 5 of gestation (Fig. 1.36). The thymus gland is formed by week 8, and is fully differentiated and producing viable lymphocytes by week 17. The third pharyngeal pouch also gives rise to the parathyroid glands. Lymphoid stem cells are produced by the fetal liver and spleen, and by bone marrow from 6 months gestation.

Thymic hypoplasia

Although it continues to grow until puberty, the relative size of the thymus gland decreases over this period. After puberty there is a real reduction in size and, by adulthood, it is composed largely of adipose tissue and continues to produce far fewer T lymphocytes.

In di George syndrome, the thymus fails to develop. Consequently, there is an absence of circulating T cells and a reduction in cell-mediated immunity.

T lymphocytes
Functions of different T cell phenotypes

The different types of T cell can be differentiated by cell-surface molecules and function. There are two different types of T cell receptor (TCR), which have different functions. T cells expressing αβ-TCRs account for at least 95% of circulatory T cells. They become cytotoxic, helper or suppressor cells and, unless specified otherwise, account for all the T cells mentioned in this book. T cells expressing a γδ-TCR are present at mucosal surfaces and their specificity is biased towards certain bacterial and viral antigens. Some γδ-T cells can recognize antigen independently of an APC. These T cells are usually cytotoxic in their actions. They differ from NK cells because they detect antigen rather than the presence or absence of MHC class I molecules. They are part of the adaptive system, because their action is specific and shows evidence of immunological memory.

T helper cells

T helper (Th) cells play a key role in the development of the immune response:

- They determine the epitopes that are targeted by the immune system via their interactions with antigen in conjunction with class II MHC molecules on APCs
- They determine the nature of the immune response directed against target antigens, e.g. cytotoxic T cell response or antibody response
- They are required for normal B cell function (see p. 24).

Most Th cells are CD4[+] and can be divided into four subsets on the basis of the cytokines they secrete:

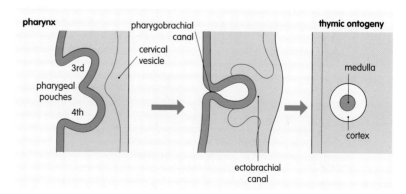

Fig. 1.36 Embryological development of the thymus. The thymus develops from the third (and possibly fourth) pharyngeal pouch. This forms the medulla, which is surrounded by the ectobranchial canal formed from the cervical vesicle. The thymus is developed by 8 weeks of gestation.

1. Th0
2. Th1
3. Th2
4. Treg.

Th0 cells arise as a result of initial short-term stimulation of naïve T cells; they are capable of secreting a broad spectrum of cytokines. Prolonged stimulation results in the emergence of Th1 and Th2 subsets. The cytokines released by the Th1 and Th2 subsets modulate one another's secretion. The different cytokine profiles of the Th1 and Th2 subsets reflect their different immunological functions (Fig. 1.37). The fourth type of helper T cell has a regulatory role. If autoreactive T cells manage to escape negative selection in the thymus, they need to be inhibited in the peripheral tissues. Regulatory T cells are capable of preventing this immune response. Their action is unknown but is thought to be via cytokines, including transforming growth factor-β, IL-5, IL-6 and IL-10.

Cytotoxic T cells
Most cytotoxic T (Tc) lymphocytes are CD8+ and recognize antigen in conjunction with class I MHC molecules (endogenous antigen). They lyse target cells via the same mechanisms as natural killer cells (see p. 10).

Development of T cells
T cell precursors are produced in the bone marrow and are transported to the thymus for development and maturation. The aim of T cell development and maturation is to select T cells with receptors that can recognize foreign antigens in conjunction with self MHC. Cells with non-functioning receptors or that are strongly self-reactive are destroyed (Fig. 1.38).

Positive selection
Positive selection occurs in the thymic cortex. T cells that are capable of binding self MHC molecules are selected. These T cells also become MHC restricted (see p. 18). Developing T cells express both CD4 and CD8 until they become MHC restricted, when either CD4 or CD8 is downregulated. They interact with class I and class II MHC molecules, on thymic epithelial cells. T cells that do not interact with the MHC molecules undergo apoptosis, as they do not receive a protective signal as a result of the TCR–MHC interaction.

Negative selection
T cells that are positively selected but have high affinity for MHC molecules and self antigen, undergo negative selection. T cells with high affinity for self MHC interact with MHC molecules on dendritic cells and macrophages and are forced to undergo apoptosis.

T cell activation
T cells are activated by interactions between the TCR and peptide bound to MHC. Activation also requires a 'second message' from the antigen-presenting cell. This process is shown in Fig. 1.39. Once T cells are activated they produce a wide range of molecules with several functions. These are primarily cytokines, which may be pro- or anti-inflammatory (see Fig. 1.37) or involved in activation of other immune cells.

Differences between Th1 and Th2 cells		
	Th1 cells	**Th2 cells**
Cytokines secreted	IL-2, IL-3, IFN-γ, TNF-β	IL-3, IL-4, IL-5, IL-10, IL-13
Functions	• responsible for classical cell-mediated immunity reactions such as delayed-type hypersensitivity and cytotoxic T cell activation • involved in responses to intracellular pathogens • activate macrophages	• promote B cell activation • involved in allergic diseases and responses to helminthic infections • induce rise in IgE and eosinophil levels

Fig. 1.37 Differences between the T helper 1 (Th1) and T helper 2 (Th2) cell subsets.

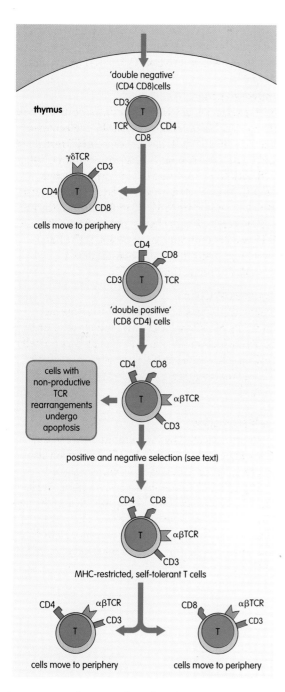

Fig. 1.38 Development of T cells in the thymus. Cells entering the thymus to become T cells are negative for CD4, CD8, CD3 and the T cell receptor (TCR). Rearrangement of the genes encoding the TCR will produce three cell lines: (1) CD4+ αβ-TCR; (2) CD8+ αβ-TCR; and (3) CD4⁻CD8⁻γδ-TCR. The β or γ chain genes rearrange first. If a functional β chain is formed, both CD4 and CD8 are upregulated and the α chain gene rearranges. The resultant T cells are positively selected if their TCR is functional, but negatively selected if they react too strongly. The majority of thymocytes will undergo apoptosis due to positive or negative selection. MHC, major histocompatibility complex.

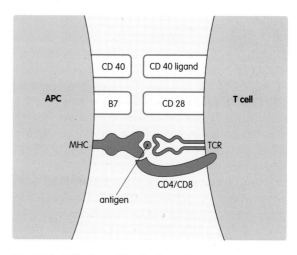

Fig. 1.39 Activation of T cells. Several interactions with antigen-presenting cells (APCs) are required to activate T cells. The T cell receptor (TCR) and CD4 or CD8 bind to MHC and antigen. CD28 on the T cell binds to B7 on the APC providing a costimulatory signal. MHC, major histocompatibility complex.

Superantigens

T cells can be activated in a non-specific fashion by superantigens. Superantigens cross-link between the V-β domain of the TCR and a class II MHC molecule on an antigen-presenting cell. Cross-linking is independent of the peptide binding cleft but depends on the framework region of the V-β domain. This means that one superantigen is able to activate about 5% of T cells, far more than normal antigen. An example of a T cell superantigen is staphylococcal enterotoxin.

Superantigens result in polyclonal activation effectively 'crowding-out' the specific, protective immune response. A consequence of polyclonal activation can be autoimmune disease. Superantigen can also result in the deletion of a large number of T cells by inducing negative selection in the thymus.

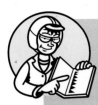

- Explain the main differences between innate and adaptive immunity.
- Explain the differences between antigen, immunogen and epitope.
- Why is immunity to protozoa and worms rare?
- What non-cellular innate barriers provide a defence against infection?
- In what ways do cells of the innate immune system combat pathogens?
- Why is pathogen killing by phagocytes accompanied by a 'respiratory burst'?
- What differences are seen between macrophages and neutrophils?
- How do natural killer (NK) cells identify virally infected and tumour cells for killing but do not kill normal cells?
- Outline the complement cascade and the actions of complement.
- What is meant by the term 'acute phase response' and what proteins are involved?
- How is recognition molecule diversity generated?
- Why don't mature lymphocytes contain the full genome?
- Neither the T cell receptor nor membrane immunoglobulin is able to signal. How do they transduce a signal?
- Why are there two classes of MHC and how does this relate to antigen presentation and cellular activation?
- What are the functions of different classes of immunoglobulins?
- How do lymphocytes recirculate and what is the relevance of this process?
- How does lymph node structure relate to function?
- What is mucosal-associated lymphoid tissue?
- What is the relevance of positive and negative selection of lymphocytes for the immune response?
- What are the differences between the different types of T helper cell?

Response to tissue damage

Inflammation is a non-specific response evoked by tissue injury. The aims of the inflammatory process are:

- Removal of the causative agent, e.g. microbes or toxins
- Removal of dead tissue
- Replacement of dead tissue with normal tissue, or scar formation.

Acute inflammation

Acute inflammation is the immediate response to cell injury. It is of short duration (a few hours to a few days) and is triggered by a range of insults, including, chemical or thermal damage and infection. Infection is sensed by resident macrophages, which release chemokines and cytokines, attracting neutrophils to the site of infection. In other instances, inflammation is initiated by resident mast cells, which tend to attract eosinophils. Once inflammation is initiated, several changes occur in vascular endothelium to allow attachment and extravasation of leucocytes—primarily neutrophils but also monocytes and lymphocytes. Attachment and extravasation requires the presence of surface molecules on both the endothelium and leucocytes. The acute inflammation process is mediated by many different chemicals.

Vascular changes

Tissue injury results in the release of chemical mediators (cytokines, chemokines and histamine) that act on local blood vessels. The main changes that occur are:

- Vasodilatation: causing increased blood flow and therefore redness and heat
- Slowing of the circulation and increased vascular permeability: formation of an inflammatory exudate results in swelling
- Entry of inflammatory cells, especially neutrophils, into the tissues.

Leucocyte extravasation

Neutrophils adhere to the vessel wall and then pass between the endothelial cells into the tissues. This is a multistep process involving:

- Margination: adherence of neutrophils to the vessel wall (Fig. 2.1)
- Diapedesis (extravasation): neutrophils move between endothelial cells into the tissue
- Chemotaxis: due to the release of several chemotactic agents (Fig. 2.2).

Integrin molecules allow immune cells to target specific sites (a process known as homing). To interact successfully with the extracellular matrix, neutrophils must express β_1-integrins, a set of adhesion molecules that can bind to collagen and laminin.

Once neutrophils reach a site of inflammation, they phagocytose foreign particles and release enzymes (see Chapter 1). Leucocytes can release proteases and metabolites during chemotaxis and phagocytosis, which are potentially harmful to the host. Neutrophils die during this process, creating pus.

Chemical mediators of inflammation

A variety of chemical mediators are produced during an inflammatory response. They usually have short half-lives and are rapidly inactivated by a variety of systems. A summary of their actions is given in Fig. 2.2.

Histamine

Histamine is released from preformed granules within mast cells, basophils and platelets. It increases vascular permeability and also causes vasodilatation.

Cell membrane phospholipid metabolites

Prostaglandins (PGs) and leukotrienes (LTs) are derived from the metabolism of arachidonic acid. Platelet-activating factor (PAF) is also an important mediator (Fig. 2.3).

Cytokines

Cytokines such as IL-8 and IL-1, and tumour necrosis factor-α (TNFα) act to:

- Induce expression of cell adhesion molecules (CAMs) on the endothelium, thus enhancing leucocyte adhesion
- Attract neutrophils to the area of injury

Margination and extravasation of neutrophils

Margination	Extravasation
Phase I 'Tethering and rolling' Weak interactions between: • L-selectin constitutively expressed on leucocytes • P- and E-selectin that are induced on endothelial cells	Further activator signals result in a conformational change in the leucocyte Metalloproteases are used to detach the cell from the endothelium, before it penetrates the endothelial basement membrane
Phase II 'Activation and strengthening' • Rapid induction of integrins on leucocytes, e.g. CD11b:CD18 (Mac-1) and CD11a:CD18 (LFA-1) on neutrophils • Integrins bind to ICAM molecules expressed constitutively on endothelial cells Phase II is mediated by chemokines	

Fig. 2.1 Margination and extravasation (diapedesis) of neutrophils. Neutrophils adhere to vessel walls via cell adhesion molecules (CAMs). CAMs can be members of the immunoglobulin gene superfamily, the selectin family or the integrin family. A variety of inflammatory mediators modify the expression or alter the affinity of CAMs. Margination is a two-phase process that is followed by cellular migration. ICAM, intercellular adhesion molecule.

Mediators of acute inflammation

Action	Mediators
Increased vascular permeability	Histamine, bradykinin, C3a, C5a, leukotrienes C_4, D_4, E_4, PAF
Vasodilation	Histamine, prostaglandins, PAF
Pain	Bradykinin, prostaglandins
Leucocyte adhesion	LTB_4, IL-1, TNF-α, C5a
Leucocyte chemotaxis	C5a, C3a, IL-8, PAF, LTB_4, fibrin and collagen fragments
Acute phase response	IL-1, TNF-α, IL-6
Tissue damage	Proteases and free radicals

Fig. 2.2 Overview of the mediators of acute inflammation. IL, interleukin; LT, leukotriene; PAF, platelet-activating factor; TNF, tumour necrosis factor.

• Induce prostacyclin (PGI_2) production
• Induce PAF synthesis
• Mediate the development of the acute phase response
• Stimulate fibroblast proliferation and increase collagen synthesis.

The complement system
This is discussed in Chapter 1.

The kinin system
Bradykinin is released following activation of the kinin system by Hageman factor (factor XII).

Bradykinin increases vascular permeability and mediates pain.

The coagulation system
The coagulation system is activated at sites of vascular injury (see p. 120). Fibrinopeptides produced during coagulation are chemotactic for neutrophils and increase vascular permeability. Thrombin also promotes fibroblast proliferation and leucocyte adhesion.

The fibrinolytic system
Plasmin (see p. 125) has several functions in the inflammatory process, including:

Fig. 2.3 Metabolism of membrane phospholipids in acute inflammation. LT, leukotriene; PAF, platelet-activating factor; PG, prostaglandin.

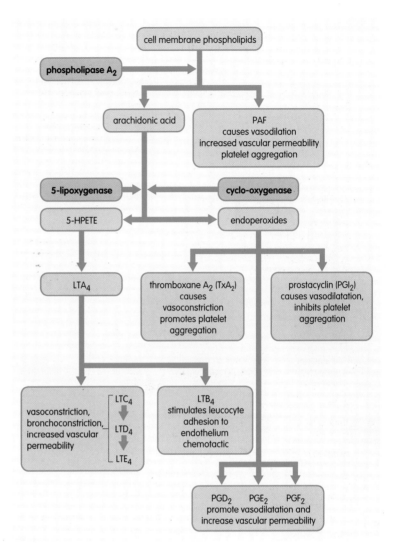

- Activation of complement via C3
- Cleavage of fibrin to form 'fibrin degradation products', which may increase vascular permeability.

Results of acute inflammation

There are several possible outcomes resulting from acute inflammation. These include:
- Regrowth and resolution
- Healing by collagenous scar formation
- Abscess formation
- Chronic inflammation.

Chronic inflammation

Chronic inflammation arises:
- When the causative agent cannot be eliminated and antigenic persistence occurs. This may be due

to deficiencies in the host response or certain microorganisms, e.g. *Mycobacterium tuberculosis*
- As a result of persistent autoimmune reactions, e.g. systemic lupus erythematosus (SLE) and rheumatoid arthritis. The body is, of course, incapable of clearing autoantigens.

The key cells of chronic inflammation are macrophages, lymphocytes and plasma cells. This is in marked contrast to acute inflammation, which is characterized primarily by a neutrophilic inflammation. Ongoing inflammation is associated with tissue destruction, but also healing.

In chronic inflammation, macrophage numbers are increased because they are recruited by chemotactic factors (e.g. platelet-derived growth factor (PDGF) and C5a) and are prevented from leaving by

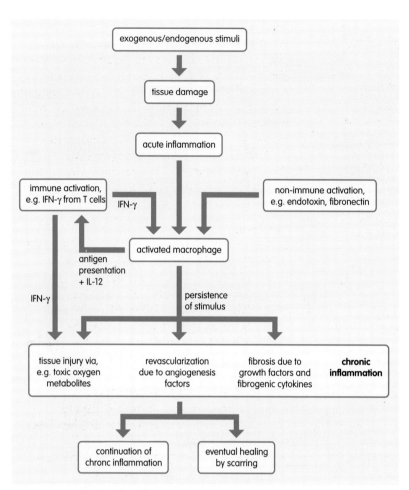

Fig. 2.4 Overview of chronic inflammation. Macrophages can be activated by T cells or by non-immune mechanisms. Activated macrophages persist at sites of chronic inflammation because of persistent stimulation. They release a number of molecules, which produce the characteristic features of chronic inflammation. Macrophages act as antigen-presenting cells to T cells, which can then activate further macrophages.

migration inhibition factor. Macrophage secretory products mediate characteristic features of chronic inflammation:

- Tissue damage via proteases and oxygen radicals
- Revascularization via angiogenic factors
- Fibroblast migration and proliferation via growth factors (e.g. PDGF) and cytokines (IL-2, TNF-α)
- Collagen synthesis via growth factors (e.g. PDGF) and cytokines (IL-1, TNF-α)
- Remodelling via collagenases
- Simulation of T cell activity by secretion of IL-12.

Lymphocytes and plasma cells are also present at the site of inflammation. In the case of chronic infections, both macrophages and T cells are required to control infection. An overview of chronic inflammation is given in Fig. 2.4.

Inflammation in disease

Inflammation is intended to protect the host but can, under certain circumstances, prove destructive. Antigenic persistence results in the continued activation and accumulation of macrophages. This leads to the formation of epithelioid cells (slightly modified macrophages) and granuloma formation (Fig. 2.5). TNF-α is needed for granuloma formation and maintenance. Interferon-γ (IFN-γ), released by activated T cells, causes macrophage transformation into epithelioid and multinucleate giant cells (which arise from the fusion of several macrophages). The granuloma is surrounded by a cuff of lymphocytes and the migration of fibroblasts results in increased collagen synthesis. Caseous necrotic areas (dry, 'cheese-like' white mass of degenerated tissue) might be present in the centre of a granuloma.

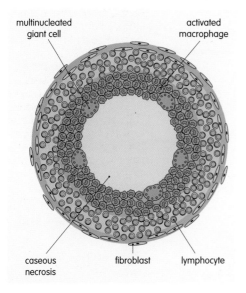

Fig. 2.5 A granuloma, showing typical focal accumulation of lymphocytes and macrophages around a central area of caseous necrosis.

The nature of the damaging stimulus determines the type of granuloma formed. Inert particles (e.g. silica in the lungs) are predominantly surrounded by macrophages. Microorganisms such as *M. tuberculosis* (which causes tuberculosis) induce a persistent, delayed-type hypersensitivity (DTH) response, resulting in granuloma formation in the lung and possibly leading to cavitation (see p. 44). The granuloma formed is characterized by focal accumulation of lymphocytes and macrophages. Phagocytosis is not usually effective because the microorganism can survive and multiply within macrophages. The granulomatous response, although preventing spread of infection, is harmful to the host.

Immune response to pathogens

Immune response to viral infection
Viruses do not always kill host cells but budding and release of new viral particles often causes the cells to lyse. The immune system can act to prevent infection, or spread of infection, or to eliminate an intracellular target once infection has occurred.

Humoral immunity to viruses
The humoral response is involved in preventing entry to, and viral replication within, cells.

Antibody
Antibodies can bind to free virus and prevent its attachment and entry to a cell (neutralization of virus particles). Antibodies can also bind to viral proteins expressed on the surface of infected cells. Antibody bound to cells can initiate antibody-dependent cell-mediated cytotoxicity (ADCC) and complement activation, and acts as an opsonin for phagocytes.

Responses directed against free virus are considered to be the most important in vivo, and antibodies are therefore important early in the course of infection to prevent spread of virus between cells.

Interferon
Interferons (IFNs) are produced by virally infected cells. IFN-α and IFN-β act on neighbouring uninfected cells and inhibit transcription and translation of viral proteins. IFN-γ activates macrophages and natural killer (NK) cells and enhances the adaptive immune response by upregulating expression of major histocompatibility complex (MHC) class I and class II molecules.

Cell-mediated immunity to viruses
Cell-mediated mechanisms are important for eliminating virus once infection is established. The cells involved include:
- NK cells: these are cytotoxic for virus-infected cells and participate in ADCC
- Cytotoxic CD8$^+$ T cells: viral peptides are presented on the cell surface in association with class I MHC molecules. CD8$^+$ T cells can destroy these infected cells
- CD4$^+$ T cell: T helper cells are required for the generation of antibody and cytotoxic T cell responses, and the recruitment and activation of macrophages (Th1 help).

An overview of the immune response to viruses is given in Fig. 2.6.

Examples of viral infection and strategies to avoid immunity
Viral infections are common and most are self-limiting. Some, particularly those that can evade the immune response, can be chronic and are potentially fatal [e.g. HIV (see p. 57) and hepatitis B]. Different viruses use different strategies to evade the host's immune response:
- Antigenic shift and drift: these are mechanisms of antigenic variation, e.g. influenza

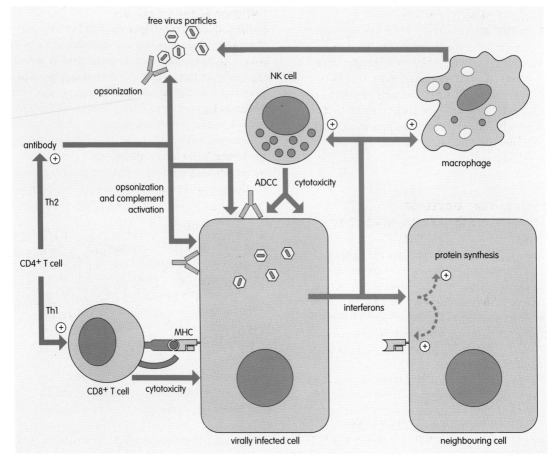

Fig. 2.6 The immune response to viruses. Interferons, produced by virally infected cells, have three important actions. Interferon-α and interferon-β induce an antiviral state in neighbouring cells (inhibition of viral transcription and translation). Interferon-γ activates macrophages and natural killer (NK) cells and upregulates major histocompatibility (MHC) molecules. NK cells kill virally infected cells either by detecting the absence of MHC class I molecules or by antibody-dependent cell-mediated cytotoxicity (ADCC). Macrophages phagocytose opsonized free virus and cell fragments, and produce further interferon. CD8+ (cytotoxic) T cells, sense viral peptides presented by MHC class I molecules and destroy the cell. CD4+ (helper) T cells help to activate macrophages and are involved in the generation of antibody and cytotoxic T cell responses.

- Polymorphism: e.g. adenovirus, rhinovirus
- Latent virus: e.g. herpes simplex virus (HSV), varicella zoster
- Modulation of MHC expression: cytomegalovirus (CMV), adenovirus, Epstein–Barr virus (EBV), HSV, HIV
- Infection of lymphocytes, e.g. HIV, measles, CMV
- Prevention of complement activation, e.g. HSV.

Antigenic variation, either by mutation or polymorphism, circumvents immunological memory because the virus expresses different immunological targets. By becoming latent, virus 'hides' from the immune system. Latent virus often reactivates when the immune system is compromised, suggesting that there must be some interaction between the immune system and the virus even when it is latent. Mechanisms that prevent normal effector functions from being carried out primarily involve downregulation of MHC class I expression. However, viruses can also interfere with IFN or produce inhibitory cytokines. Infection of lymphocytes, and their death, reduces the ability of the immune system to combat viral infection.

Immune response to bacterial infection

Bacteria are prokaryotic organisms. Their cell membrane is surrounded by a peptidoglycan cell wall. Many bacteria also have a capsule of large, branched polysaccharides. Bacteria attach to cells via surface pili, but only some bacteria enter host cells. Different immune mechanisms operate, depending on whether the bacteria are extracellular or intracellular.

Extracellular bacteria
Humoral immunity to extracellular bacteria
Complement

Bacteria activate complement via the lectin or alternative pathways. Activated complement products play a role in the elimination of bacteria, especially C3b (an opsonin), C3a and C5a (anaphylatoxins that recruit leucocytes), and the membrane attack complex (MAC), which can perforate the outer lipid bilayer of Gram-negative bacteria.

Lysozyme

Lysozyme is a naturally occurring antibacterial that attacks N-acetyl muramic acid-N-acetyl glucosamine links in the bacterial cell wall. This results in bacterial lysis.

Antibody

This is the principal defence against extracellular bacteria:
- sIgA binds to bacteria and prevents their binding to epithelial cells
- Antibody neutralizes bacterial toxins
- Antibody activates complement
- Antibody acts as an opsonin.

Cell-mediated immunity to extracellular bacteria

Phagocytic cells kill most bacteria; C3b and antibody enhance phagocytosis. Bacterial antigens are processed and presented, in conjunction with class II MHC molecules, on the surface of APCs, to CD4+ T cells. CD4+ T cell help is required for the generation of the antibody response (Th2 help).

An overview of the immune response to extracellular bacteria is given in Fig. 2.7.

Intracellular bacteria
Humoral immunity to intracellular bacteria

The humoral mechanisms that are employed against extracellular bacteria will be used to try to prevent bacteria causing intracellular infection. However, they will not be effective once the infection is intracellular.

Cell-mediated immunity to intracellular bacteria

Cell-mediated immunity is very important in the defence against intracellular bacterial infections, such as those caused by *M. tuberculosis*:
- Macrophages attempt to phagocytose the bacteria. If the organisms persist, chronic inflammation will ensue. This can lead to delayed (type IV) hypersensitivity (see p. 50)
- Cells infected with bacteria can activate NK cells, which cause cytotoxicity and can activate macrophages
- CD4+ T cells release cytokines that activate macrophages (Th1 help)

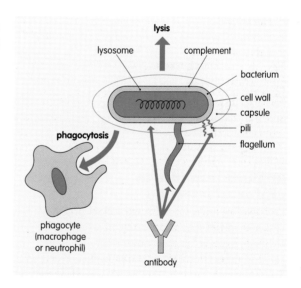

Fig. 2.7 The immune response to extracellular bacteria. The first line of host defence against bacteria is lysozyme. This 'natural antibiotic' attacks N-acetyl muramic acid-N-acetyl glucosamine links in the bacterial cell wall. This, together with complement, leads to bacterial lysis. Antibody is produced against flagella (immobilizing) and pili (prevents attachment). Capsular polysaccharides can induce T-cell-independent antibody. Antibodies aid complement activation and phagocytosis of bacteria.

- CD8$^+$ T cells recognize antigens presented in conjunction with class I MHC molecules on the surface of infected cells and lyse these cells.

Examples of infection and bacterial strategies to avoid immunity

Bacterial strategies to avoid the immune response must allow one of the following:
- Prevent phagocytosis
- Allow survival within phagocytes
- Prevent complement activation
- Avoid recognition by the immune system.

Strategies to avoid immunity include:
- Capsules can inhibit phagocytosis, e.g. *Streptococcus pneumoniae*, *Haemophilus* spp.
- Killing of phagocytes by toxins, e.g. *Staphylococcus* spp.
- Neutralization of opsonizing IgG, e.g. *Staphylococcus* spp.
- Survival within phagocytes, e.g. *M. tuberculosis*, *Mycobacterium leprae*, *Toxoplasma* spp.
- Inhibition of complement activation, e.g. *Staphylococcus* spp., *Streptococcus* spp., *Haemophilus* spp., *Pseudomonas* spp.
- Polymorphism, e.g. *Streptococcus pneumoniae*, *Salmonella typhi*.

Like viruses, bacteria can be highly polymorphic. Bacteria of the same species can appear to be entirely different to the immune system.

Immune response to protozoal infection

Protozoa are microscopic, single-celled organisms. Fewer than 20 types of protozoa infect man, although malaria, trypanosomes and *Leishmania* cause significant morbidity and mortality. Protozoa cause intracellular infection, have marked antigenic variation and are often immunosuppressive. They have complex lifecycles, with several different stages, and therefore present the immune system with a variety of challenges. Protozoal infection is often chronic, as the immune system is not very efficient at dealing with these organisms. Most of the pathology of protozoal disease is caused by the immune response.

Humoral immunity against protozoa

Complement and antibody are important during the extracellular stage of infection. This opsonizes the protozoa and can cause lysis or prevent infection.

Cell-mediated immunity against protozoa
- **Phagocytosis:** by macrophages, monocytes and neutrophils is an important part of the immune response against protozoa
- **CD4$^+$ T cells:** are activated in response to protozoal infection. The subset of CD4$^+$ T cells activated is thought to determine whether the immune response is protective or not. T helper 1 cytokines, e.g. IL-2, IFN-γ, TNF-β, are considered protective
- **Cytotoxic CD8$^+$ T cells:** are important in destroying protozoa that replicate within cells, e.g. the sporozoite stage of *Plasmodium falciparum* (which causes malaria)
- **NK cells and mast cells:** are often activated in protozoal infection.

Examples of protozoal infection and evasion of the immune response

Protozoa have good mechanisms to prevent the initiation of an immune response. Strategies include:
- Escape into the cytoplasm following phagocytosis, e.g. *Trypanosoma cruzi*
- Prevention of complement actions, e.g. *Leishmania* spp.
- Gene switching to create antigen variation, e.g. trypanosomes
- Immunosuppression, e.g. trypanosomes.

Hypersensitivity mechanisms

Concepts of hypersensitivity

Hypersensitivity is an exaggerated or inappropriate immune response that causes tissue damage (immunopathology). The antigens involved are often innocuous. The mechanisms used to eliminate antigen under normal circumstances can cause damage to normal tissues (hypersensitivity). Hypersensitivity can take place in response to:
- An infection that cannot be cleared, e.g. tuberculosis
- A normally harmless exogenous substance, e.g. pollen
- An autoantigen, e.g. DNA in SLE.

Hypersensitivity reactions have been classified, by Gell and Coombs, into four types: I, II, III, and IV. Types I, II, and III are antibody-mediated; type IV is cell-mediated.

Type I hypersensitivity

In type I (or immediate) hypersensitivity, the antigen (allergen) induces a humoral IgE immune response. On first exposure to the allergen, an individual produces specific IgE. IgE binds to high-affinity Fc-ε receptors (receptors for the Fc portion of the IgE molecule) on mast cells and basophils. Upon subsequent exposures, cross-linking of membrane-bound IgE induces release of preformed and newly synthesized mediators. Their effects can be localized or systemic (see p. 12). The immune mechanisms of type I reactions are illustrated in Fig. 2.8. Examples of type I reactions include:

- Allergic rhinitis (hayfever): pollens
- Allergic asthma: house-dust mite
- Systemic anaphylaxis: penicillin, peanuts or insect venom.

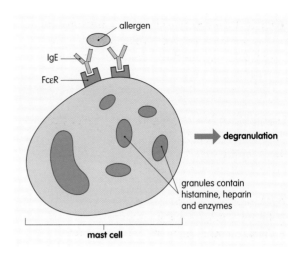

Fig. 2.8 The immune mechanisms of type I hypersensitivity reactions. Cross-linkage of IgE bound to cell surface receptors on mast cells and basophils results in degranulation.

Atopy is a genetic predisposition to produce IgE in response to many common, naturally occurring allergens. It has a prevalence of 10–30%. Atopic patients can suffer from multiple allergies. The genetic basis of atopy is not known.

Diagnosis of type I reactions is by the skin-prick test, in which a number of allergens are applied to adjacent areas of the skin of the forearm. In type I hypersensitivity, a wheal-and-flare reaction occurs within 15 minutes. Serum IgE levels (total and specific for a particular allergen) are also used to assess type I hypersensitivity, when skin-prick testing is unsafe. Specific IgE can be detected by a radio-allergo-sorbent test (RAST). A number of antigens are bound to a paper disc, to which the serum to be tested is added. Specific IgE that binds to the antigen is subsequently bound by radiolabelled anti-human IgE antibodies.

Type II hypersensitivity

Type II (or cytotoxic) hypersensitivity occurs when antibody specific for cell surface antigens is produced. Cell destruction can then result via:
- Complement activation
- Antibody-dependent cell-mediated cytotoxicity (ADCC)
- Phagocytosis.

The immune mechanisms of type II hypersensitivity reactions are summarized in Fig. 2.9.

Examples of type II reactions in which complement is activated and cells destroyed are:
- Incompatible blood transfusions
- Haemolytic disease of the newborn
- Autoimmune haemolytic anaemias.

Several diseases are caused by antibody directed against cell surface receptors, which can stimulate or block the receptor. In Graves' disease, stimulating antibodies are directed against the receptor for thyroid stimulating hormone. In myasthenia gravis, antibodies are directed against the acetylcholine receptor. They can destroy the receptor or cause lysis due to complement activation.

Type III hypersensitivity

In type III (or immune-complex-mediated) hypersensitivity, antibody combines with soluble

43

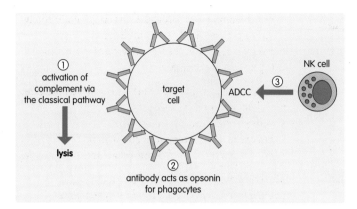

Fig. 2.9 The immune mechanisms of type II hypersensitivity reactions. Antibody bound to cells (either antibody to foreign cells or autoantibody) results in cell death via (1) complement, (2) phagocytes or (3) natural killer (NK) cells. ADCC, antibody-dependent cell-mediated cytotoxicity.

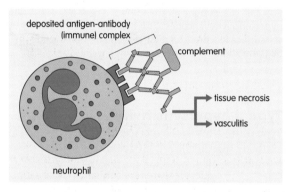

Fig. 2.10 The immune mechanisms of type III hypersensitivity reactions. Immune complexes that are normally removed by phagocytes are deposited in blood vessels or the tissues resulting in severe damage via complement and neutrophils.

antigen. The resulting immune complexes are usually phagocytosed but, if they persist, can cause immune complex disease (Fig. 2.10).

The immune complexes can be deposited in tissues near the site of antigen entry (localized type III reaction). This is demonstrated by the Arthus reaction, in which an intradermal or subcutaneous injection of antigen into a recipient with high levels of appropriate circulating antibody produces localized immune complexes that activate complement and generate acute inflammation.

Localized type III reactions are exemplified by:
• Farmer's lung: repeated inhalation of actinomycetes found in mouldy hay
• Pigeon-fancier's disease: repeated inhalation of antigens found in dried pigeon faeces.

If immune complexes form in blood, they circulate around the body and are deposited in the blood vessel walls of a number of tissues, especially the kidneys and joints (generalized type III reaction). Systemic type III reactions can cause autoimmune diseases such as SLE and occur in infectious diseases such as malaria and viral hepatitis.

Type IV hypersensitivity

Upon first contact with antigen, a subset of CD4+ T helper (Th) cells is activated and clonally expanded (this takes 1–2 weeks). Upon subsequent encounter with the same antigen, sensitized Th cells secrete cytokines. These attract and activate macrophages, which account for more than 95% of the cells involved. Activated macrophages have increased phagocytic ability and can destroy pathogens more effectively. The type IV reaction peaks at 48–72 hours after contact with the antigen (time taken for the recruitment and activation of the macrophages) and is therefore known as delayed-type hypersensitivity. An overview of the immune mechanisms involved is given in Fig. 2.11.

Type IV reactions are important for the clearance of intracellular pathogens. However, if antigen persists, the response can be detrimental to the individual, as the lytic products of the activated macrophages can damage healthy tissues. Examples of antigens that induce a type IV response are:
• Contact antigens such as nickel and poison ivy
• Intracellular pathogens such as *M. tuberculosis* and *Leishmania major*.

Skin testing is performed to detect type IV reactions. The tuberculin skin test can be used to determine

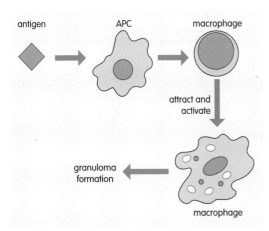

Fig. 2.11 The immune mechanisms of type IV hypersensitivity reactions. These reactions take several days to be initiated because antigen is first presented to T cells, which can then activate macrophages. APC, antigen-presenting cells.

whether a person has been exposed to *M. tuberculosis*. An intradermal injection of purified protein derivative (PPD) is given to the individual. Previous exposure to *M. tuberculosis* or bacille Calmette–Guérin (BCG) vaccination results in a positive response. This is apparent as a firm red (due to the intense infiltration of macrophages) lesion at the injection site 48–72 hours after the injection.

Anti-inflammatory drugs

Anti-inflammatory drugs are used commonly for the treatment of a variety of conditions. Different types of anti-inflammatory drug are available including:
- Steroids
- Non-steroidal anti-inflammatory drugs
- Other anti-inflammatory agents.

Steroids
The adrenal cortex releases several steroid hormones into the circulation. Glucocorticoids affect carbohydrate and protein metabolism, but also have effects on the immune system acting as immunosuppressive and anti-inflammatory agents. Several glucocorticoids are available therapeutically, including:
- Hydrocortisone: can be given intravenously in status asthmaticus or topically for inflammatory skin conditions

- Prednisolone: oral preparations are given in many inflammatory or allergic conditions
- Beclomethasone: used as an aerosol in asthma or topically for eczema.

Conditions commonly treated with steroids include:
- Inflammatory bowel disease
- Allergic conditions, e.g. asthma
- Severe inflammatory skin conditions
- Severe inflammatory rheumatological conditions.

Steroids act by entering cells, particularly macrophages, where they bind receptors and stimulate the transcription of hundreds of genes. Suppression of inflammation is by a variety of mechanisms:
- Reduction in the number of circulating lymphocytes and macrophages
- Inhibition of phospholipase A_2 and therefore the formation of pro-inflammatory arachidonic acid metabolites
- Inhibition of complement.

Adverse effects and contraindications
Glucocorticoids cause many adverse effects at the high doses required to produce an anti-inflammatory effect. The clinical features are similar to those seen in Cushing's syndrome and the adverse effects are shown in Fig. 2.12. Steroids are contraindicated if there is evidence of systemic infection. Long-term high dose steroid therapy is usually avoided.

Non-steroidal anti-inflammatory drugs (NSAIDs)
NSAIDs include a large number of drugs that can be bought over the counter, e.g. aspirin and paracetamol. They are chemically diverse but all act to inhibit cyclo-oxygenase (Fig. 2.13). This attenuates, but does not abolish, inflammation. As well as their anti-inflammatory effects, NSAIDs have analgesic and antipyretic actions. They are used primarily in conditions where pain is accompanied by inflammation, such as rheumatoid arthritis.

Aspirin
Acetylsalicylic acid (aspirin) is anti-inflammatory but causes a lot of adverse effects. As a consequence of this, newer NSAIDs (e.g. ibuprofen) are usually preferred for treatment of inflammatory conditions, because they exhibit fewer side-effects.

Adverse effects of glucocorticoids	
Body System	**Symptoms**
Gastrointestinal	Dyspepsia, nausea, peptic ulceration, abdominal distension, acute pancreatitis, oesophageal ulceration, candidiasis
Musculoskeletal	Proximal myopathy, osteoporosis, avascular osteonecrosis
Endocrine	Adrenal suppression, menstrual irregularities, hirsutism, weight gain, negative nitrogen and calcium balance, increased appetite, increased susceptibility to infection
Neuropsychiatric	Euphoria, psychological dependence, depression, insomnia, aggravation of epilepsy, psychosis
Ophthalmic	Glaucoma, papilloedema, cataracts
Skin	Impaired wound healing, atrophy, easy bruising, striae, telangectasia, acne

Fig. 2.12 The adverse effects of glucocorticoids.

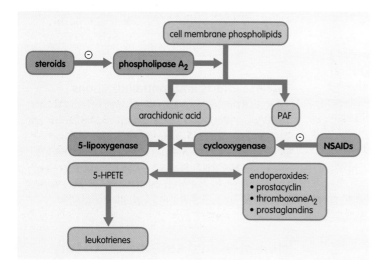

Fig. 2.13 The actions of non-steroidal anti-inflammatory drugs (NSAIDs) in arachidonic acid metabolism. PAF, platelet-activating factor.

Paracetamol

Paracetamol has good analgesic properties but little effect on inflammation.

Adverse effects and contraindications

Adverse effects with NSAIDs are common. They often cause damage to the mucosa of the gastrointestinal tract because they remove the cytoprotective effects of prostaglandins in the gut; the mucosa becomes ulcerated because of the damaging effects of stomach acid. Many NSAID preparations, e.g. enteric-coating, are designed to reduce ulceration. NSAIDs can also be nephrotoxic and cause bronchospasm. Side-effects of aspirin include nausea, vomiting, epigastric pain and tinnitus.

Other anti-inflammatory drugs

Other anti-inflammatory drugs reduce inflammation via different mechanisms. These include:

- Immunosuppressive drugs, such as ciclosporin and azathioprine (main effects on T cells)
- Methotrexate (main effects on macrophages).

Such drugs are often used in chronic inflammatory conditions, e.g. rheumatoid arthritis, to reduce the need for steroids. Each drug has specific adverse effects and contraindications. Newer approaches use biological agents to block the effects of pro-inflammatory cytokines. For example, the effects of TNF can be blocked by infliximab (monoclonal anti-TNF) or etanercept (soluble TNF receptor). Both drugs are very effective in the treatment of rheumatoid arthritis and Crohn's disease. However, they can increase the risk of infections, such as tuberculosis, in which TNF normally has a protective role.

Investigation of immune function

Electrophoresis

Electrophoresis uses an electric field to separate proteins or nucleic acids on the basis of size, electric charge and other physical properties. An electric current is passed across a support matrix (e.g. cellulose acetate, polyacrylamide gel) or a solution. As particles travel at different rates (because of their different electrical charge and size), they gradually separate to form bands, which can be visualized by staining. Electrophoresis is commonly used to detect excess light-chain protein in multiple myeloma (see p. 109).

Flow cytometry and immunofluoresence

Flow cytometry is a useful tool for differentiating between different populations of cells, as well as for counting the number of cells within a sample. This is done by producing a very fine stream of medium, where only one cell at a time passes through a beam of laser light. Sensors detect when a cell blocks the beam of light and the amount of light scatter identifies the size and granularity of the cell. Various surface antigens on the cell can be bound by monoclonal antibodies (specific for one antigen). The monoclonal antibodies are labelled with dyes that fluoresce under laser light (immunofluoresence). Different types of dye allow the detection of specific antigens (most machines use red and green fluorescence, but up to five colours are used by some machines).

Immunoassays

These use specific antibody to detect antigen (which might itself be an antibody). Different types of immunoassay use different forms of labelling.

ELISA

Enzyme-linked immunosorbent assay (ELISA) uses enzyme reactions to identify the presence of antigen. In ELISA, the ligand that binds to the test antibody is covalently coupled to an enzyme (e.g. peroxidase), which converts a colourless substrate into a coloured product. The density of colour relates to the amount of antigen (Fig. 2.14). ELISA is usually used to measure antibody to specific antigen. In this case, the

Fig. 2.14 Enzyme-linked immunosorbent assay (ELISA). ELISA can be used to detect antigens but is most commonly used to measure antibody to specific antigen (e.g. a virus) and this is shown. Viral antigen is bound to a plate and the patient's serum added. If specific IgG is present it will bind to the antigen. Enzyme labelled anti-IgG is added (binding to the patient's IgG). The enzyme converts a colourless substrate into a coloured product. The intensity of colour is relative to the amount of antigen.

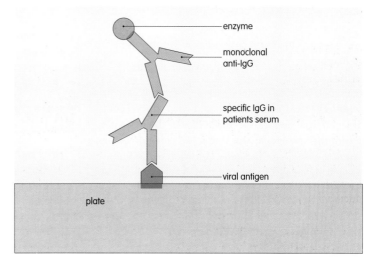

patient's serum will be added to a plate that has antigen bound to it. The presence of specific IgG can then be detected.

Radioimmunoassays
Radioisotopes were a commonly used label in immunoassays, however, fluorescent or chemiluminescent labelling is safer and is replacing the use of radioisotopes.

Coombs test
Coombs reagent is a preparation of antibodies, raised in animals, directed against one of the following:
- Human immunoglobulin
- Complement
- Specific immunoglobulin, e.g. anti-human IgG.

The direct Coombs test
This is used to detect antibody or complement already bound to the red cells. A positive direct Coombs test is found in:
- Autoimmune haemolytic anaemias
- Alloimmune haemolytic anaemias (haemolytic disease of the newborn and transfusion reactions)
- Drug-induced immune haemolytic anaemias.

The indirect Coombs test
This is used to detect antibody in the serum. It can be used in the following situations:
- Routine cross-matching of blood prior to transfusion
- Detection of blood group antibodies in pregnancy
- Detection of serum antibodies in autoimmune haemolytic anaemias.

In cross-matching of blood, serum from the patient requiring transfusion is incubated with the red cells of a potential donor. Any antibodies in the patient's serum that are specific for donor red cell antigens interact with donor red cells. Addition of Coombs reagent then causes agglutination of the red cells, as described for the direct Coombs test.

Testing phagocyte function
The numbers of neutrophils can be detected on a full blood count (see p. 131). Neutrophil function is tested by a nitroblue tetrazolium (NBT) reduction test. Following activation of neutrophils, the metabolic burst accompanies the production of many reactive chemicals, including superoxide and hydrogen peroxide. These chemicals, which cause intracellular killing, are able to reduce NBT, a blue dye. Failure of reduction is present in chronic granulomatous disease (see Fig. 2.24).

Testing cell-mediated immunity
An intradermal injection of antigen (e.g. the Mantoux test for tuberculosis) or skin-patch testing (e.g. to nickel) can detect cell-mediated type IV hypersensitivity. T cell function can be monitored, e.g. during immunosuppressive therapy, by looking at responses to mitogens.

Tests for autoimmunity
The presence of autoantibodies can be detected in many rheumatic and endocrine disorders. Rheumatoid factor (RF), commonly seen in rheumatoid arthritis (see p. 52), is an anti-IgG antibody. However, RF is not always present in rheumatoid arthritis and can occur in other rheumatic conditions. It can be detected by agglutination of latex particles or sheep red blood cells that have been coated with immunoglobulin.

Indirect immunofluoresence of a range of tissues can be used to detect autoantibodies to nuclear and cytoplasmic antigens. Specific antibodies, e.g. anti-double-stranded DNA in SLE (for other examples, see pp. 53 and 54), can be detected by ELISA or radioimmunoassays.

Tests for allergy
See hypersensitivity (p. 42).

Allergy
Allergy is due to hypersensitivity reactions to exogenous antigens (known as allergens), mediated by IgE. Allergic symptoms usually result from degranulation of mast cells. This process is mediated by the cross-linking of IgE by allergen. Allergic conditions are therefore type I hypersensitivity reactions. Other types of hypersensitivity cause chronic forms of allergy. The symptoms of different

allergies affect different tissues and can be local or generalized.

Asthma

Asthma is a chronic inflammatory disorder of the airways, characterized by reversible airflow obstruction. The airways become hyper-responsive and exaggerated bronchoconstriction follows a wide variety of stimuli, e.g. exercise or cold air. The symptoms of asthma are cough, wheeze, chest tightness and shortness of breath. Asthma is a common disease and is diagnosed in 5–10% of children. The incidence has risen over the last few decades, particularly in more economically developed countries.

Pollens, house-dust mite faeces and animal fur are the most common allergens. These cause inflammation of the bronchial wall involving:

- Infiltration by eosinophils, mast cells, lymphocytes and neutrophils
- Oedema of the submucosa
- Smooth muscle hypertrophy and hyperplasia
- Thickening of the basement membrane
- Mucous plugging
- Epithelial desquamation.

Asthma is diagnosed by a reversal in airway obstruction (measured by forced expiratory volume in the first second) of more than or equal to 15% following the administration of an inhaled β_2-adrenoreceptor agonist (such as salbutamol). This treatment is used for the short-term improvement of symptoms, although inhaled steroids and other immunosuppressive/anti-inflammatory drugs are used prophylactically to prevent asthma attacks.

Atopic/allergic eczema

Eczema or dermatitis can be caused by an allergic response. Dermatitis means skin inflammation. There are several types of dermatitis, including allergic eczema and contact dermatitis (a type IV hypersensitivity reaction). Allergic contact eczema (contact dermatitis) is caused by DTH. The reaction occurs wherever the allergen contacts the skin, but it can persist indefinitely. Contact dermatitis can be diagnosed by patch testing and treatment is primarily by avoidance of the allergen.

Atopic eczema is most commonly the result of exposure to pollen or house-dust mite faeces. Common allergens are shown in Fig. 2.15. About 10% of children are diagnosed with eczema. Eczema

Fig. 2.15 Summary of allergic reactions.

Allergic reactions		
Allergic condition	**Common allergens**	**Features**
Systemic anaphylaxis	Drugs Serum Venoms Peanuts	Oedema with increased vascular permeability Leads to tracheal occlusion, circulatory collapse and possibly death
Acute urticaria	Insect bites	Local wheal and flare (red and raised)
Allergic rhinitis	Pollen (hay fever) Dust-mite faeces (perennial rhinitis)	Oedema and irritation of nasal mucosa
Asthma	Pollen Dust-mite faeces	Bronchial constriction, increased mucus production, airway inflammation
Food	Shellfish Milk Eggs Fish Wheat	Itching urticaria and potentially anaphylaxis
Atopic eczema	Pollen Dust-mite faeces Some foods	Itchy inflammation of the dermis and epidermis Usually red and sometimes vesicular

commonly affects the flexural creases and the fronts of the wrist and ankles. In infancy and adulthood the face and trunk are often involved. The skin lesions are itchy, red, sometimes vesicular and might be dry. Because of itching, the skin is often excoriated, which can lead to lichenification (thickening of the skin). Eczema is often complicated by superinfection with bacteria, particularly *Staphylococcus aureus*.

The diagnosis of atopic eczema is usually clinical. Total serum IgE, RAST for specific IgE and prick testing with common allergens are occasionally performed to confirm the diagnosis of atopic eczema. Treatment of eczema is mainly topical, except in more severe cases, when systemic steroids and immunosuppressants are used. Therapies include:

- Emollients: moisturizes dry skin and reduces itching
- Topical steroids: anti-inflammatory
- Topical antibiotics or antiseptics: in infected eczema
- Oral antihistamine: reduces itching
- Ciclosporin: resistant cases might require immunosuppression.

Allergic rhinitis

Nasal congestion, watery nasal discharge and sneezing occur after exposure to allergen. The most common allergens are grass, flower, weed or tree pollens, which cause a seasonal rhinitis (hay fever), and house-dust mite faeces, which can cause a more perennial rhinitis. Allergic attacks usually last for a few hours and are often accompanied by smarting and watering of the eyes. Skin-prick tests can identify the allergen.

Treatment is with antihistamines, steroids (nasal or ocular) or mast cell stabilizers such as sodium cromoglicate. Avoidance of allergens is advised but is often difficult.

Anaphylaxis

Anaphylaxis is a medical emergency and can be fatal. However, it is rapidly reversible if treated properly. A systemic response to an allergen that is either intravenous or rapidly absorbed can cause tracheal occlusion and shock. Many allergens can cause anaphylaxis, but more common causes include drugs, bee stings and peanuts. The signs of anaphylaxis are principally those of shock. Signs include:

- Hypotension with tachycardia
- Warm peripheral temperature
- Signs of airway obstruction
- Laryngeal and facial oedema and urticaria (often seen).

The initial management of anaphylaxis is resuscitation. Allergens should be removed if possible, e.g. stop drug infusion, and the patient should be given high-flow oxygen. Adrenaline (epinephrine) should be given intramuscularly and repeated after 5 minutes if there is no improvement. Adrenaline should be given intravenously only in life-threatening profound shock. Fluids might be needed for patients in shock and a β_2-adrenreceptor agonist can be used to reverse bronchospasm. People who have had anaphylactic reactions often carry adrenaline with them so that it can be administered rapidly in an emergency. Steroids and antihistamines act too slowly to be effective in anaphylaxis.

Autoimmunity

Prevention of autoimmunity

Autoimmunity is a state in which the body exhibits immunological reactivity to itself. 'Self tolerance' is the generic term given to the mechanisms by which T and B cells are prevented from responding to self. Because T and B cells randomly recombine the genes for their receptors, there is a risk of producing receptors that will react with self antigen. These cells must be eliminated to make the host tolerant to itself.

Central tolerance

Central tolerance is by negative selection—early clonal deletion. T cells (in the thymus) and B cells (in the bone marrow) are eliminated if they are self reactive. Central tolerance is not complete. Only the most self-reactive lymphocytes are deleted, ensuring that a wide lymphocyte repertoire is maintained.

Peripheral tolerance

In the periphery, self antigens do not generally elicit an immune response. Several mechanisms prevent self-reactive T cells from causing autoimmune disease, including:

- Lack of the co-stimulatory molecules required for T cell activation, e.g. cells expressing self antigen do not express CD40 or CD28
- Sequestration of the antigen behind a physical barrier, e.g. the testis
- Lack of antigen presentation
- T cells entering immune privileged sites undergo apoptosis (via Fas, transforming growth factor (TGF)-β or IL-10). Immune privileged sites include the brain, testis and the anterior chamber of the eye
- A negative feedback system (cytotoxic T lymphocyte antigen 4) prevents over-stimulation of an immune response.

Immune regulation
Response to self antigen can also be regulated by a population of T cells producing suppressive cytokines. Regulatory T cells inhibit responses of other T cells through mechanisms that are as yet poorly understood.

Causes of autoimmunity— breakdown of tolerance
If tolerance breaks down, autoimmunity can develop. Tolerance can break down in the thymus (usually for genetic reasons) or in the periphery (usually as a result of environmental factors such as infection). Autoimmunity is multifactorial, a defect in at least one of the regulatory mechanisms is required before disease develops.

Role of human leucocyte antigen (HLA)—genetic predisposition
Many autoimmune diseases have a familial component. The HLA haplotype is the main identified genetic factor. The haplotype can influence susceptibility to developing autoimmunity via molecular mimicry. Certain HLA alleles are linked to specific autoimmune processes, e.g. HLA-DR4 in rheumatoid arthritis. However, a certain HLA haplotype does not automatically result in the development of an autoimmune disease; 95% of patients with ankylosing spondylitis have HLA-B27, but only 5% of the population with HLA-B27 have ankylosing spondylitis.

Release of sequestered antigens
Sequestered antigens are not seen by the developing immune system and therefore they are not deleted centrally. Tissue trauma can release previously sequestered antigen into the circulation, and an immune response can develop as a consequence.

Role of infection—molecular mimicry
Certain bacteria and viruses possess antigens that resemble sequestered host-cell components, and infection with these can generate an immune response against self. An example of molecular mimicry is cross-reactivity between heart muscle and streptococcal antigens, leading to rheumatic fever. This is short-lived and reversible.

Role of infection—polyclonal activation
Some viral infections are able to activate B cells in a non-specific fashion. This results in the proliferation of several B cell clones, which can produce autoreactive autoantibody.

Role of HLA—inappropriate MHC expression
Upregulation of MHC class II molecules can result in activation of autoreactive T cells. Healthy β cells in the islets of Langerhans have been shown to express low levels of class I and II MHC molecules, whereas cells in individuals with insulin-dependent diabetes mellitus (IDDM) express high levels of both.

Mechanisms of autoimmunity
Autoimmune diseases are hypersensitivity reactions in which an exaggerated response is triggered by self antigen. Autoimmune diseases can therefore be classified in the same way as hypersensitivity.

Antibody-mediated (type II hypersensitivity reactions)
Antibodies that are specific for self antigen bind to tissues or cells. Autoimmunity can result from a variety of mechanisms, including:
- Opsonization: e.g. autoimmune haemolytic anaemia, IgG binds to red blood cells, which are phagocytosed by macrophages in the spleen
- Complement activation: e.g. in severe autoimmune haemolytic anaemia, IgM antibodies bound to red blood cells activate complement, resulting in lysis within the circulation.

Neutralization and ADCC can also occur in response to self antigen.

Immune-complex-mediated (type III hypersensitivity reactions)

Immune complexes are lattices of antigen and antibody. They are usually cleared rapidly from the circulation, but complexes that are not cleared trigger inflammation, particularly in blood vessels. An example of a type III autoimmune disease is SLE. A consequence of the presence of circulating immune complexes can be the development of glomerulonephritis. Immune complexes deposit in the capillaries of the glomerular tufts in the kidneys, resulting in renal failure. Immune complexes are also deposited at other sites, e.g. joints.

Cell-mediated (type IV hypersensitivity reactions)

These comprise autoimmune T cell responses, usually by T helper and T cytotoxic cells. Examples include rheumatoid arthritis and type I diabetes mellitus.

Systemic autoimmune diseases
Systemic lupus erythematosus (SLE)

In SLE, autoantibodies can be directed against DNA, histone proteins, red blood cells, platelets, leucocytes and clotting factors. Diagnosis is by antinuclear antibody testing. It is most commonly diagnosed in women in the second or third decade of life.

The aetiology is unknown but the vast array of autoantibodies present suggests a breakdown of self tolerance. Genetic factors predispose to the disease. There is an association with HLA-DR2 and HLA-DR3, and with deficiencies of complement proteins, especially C2 or C4. Other relevant aetiological factors include drugs such as hydralazine and exposure to ultraviolet light.

Deposition of immune complexes leads to the various clinical features of SLE, including:
- Arthritis (deposition in joints)
- Rashes in sun exposed areas
- Glomerulonephritis.

SLE is treated with immunosuppression, steroids, NSAIDs or other anti-inflammatory drugs.

Rheumatoid arthritis (RA)

RA is a chronic systemic disease that primarily involves the joints, resulting in inflammation of the synovium and destruction of the articular cartilage (Fig. 2.16). Initially, the disease affects the small joints of the hands and feet symmetrically, later spreading to the larger joints. RA affects approximately 1–2% of the world's population and is most common between the ages of 30 and 55 years. The female:male ratio is 3:1.

Approximately 70% of RA patients carry either the HLA-DR4 or HLA-DR1 haplotype. The

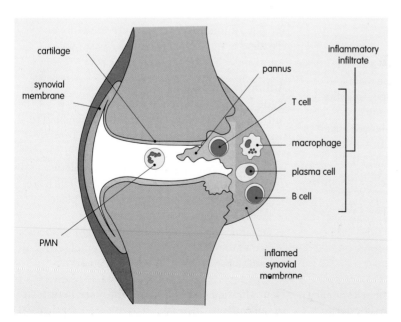

Fig. 2.16 Rheumatoid joint showing pannus formation and cartilage destruction. The synovial membrane is infiltrated by inflammatory cells, and hypertrophies to form granulation tissue known as 'pannus'. This eventually erodes the articular cartilage and bone. T cells and macrophages in the inflamed synovium secrete tumour necrosis factor. PMN, polymorphonuclear neutrophil.

Fig. 2.17 Pathogenesis of rheumatoid arthritis (RA). Autoreactive CD4+ T cells mediate the pathological changes. Synovial T cells produce a number of cytokines including tumour necrosis factor (TNF). These stimulate the acute phase response, synovial inflammation and bone erosion. Activation of B cells can result in the production of rheumatoid factor and immune complex formation.

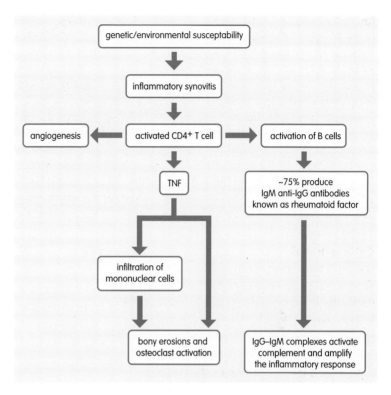

immunopathogenesis of RA is outlined in Fig. 2.17. A key event in RA is secretion of TNF by T cells and macrophages. TNF causes joint inflammation and erosion of bone, and can be blocked by infliximab.

A summary of other systemic connective tissue disorders and vasculitidies is given in Figs 2.18 and 2.19.

Organ- or cell-type-specific autoimmune disease

A summary of organ- or cell-type-specific diseases is given in Fig. 2.20.

Hashimoto's thyroiditis

Hashimoto's thyroiditis is the most common cause of goitrous hypothyroidism. Antigen-specific cytotoxic T cells attack the thyroid gland, leading to progressive destruction of the epithelium. Marked lymphocytic infiltration (mainly by B cells and CD4+ T cells) of the thyroid gland is accompanied by migration of large numbers of macrophages and plasma cells, resulting in the formation of lymphoid follicles and germinal centres within the thyroid. Due to unregulated T-helper cell interaction with

B cells, autoantibodies are produced against thyroid antigens such as thyroid peroxidase.

Middle-aged females are most commonly affected (female:male ratio of 5:1). The disease is associated with HLA-DR5 and HLA-DR3 haplotypes.

Graves' disease

The disease is characterized by hyperthyroidism. This is thought to arise as a result of IgG autoantibody production against parts of the thyroid stimulating hormone receptor. Clinical features include ophthalmopathy and pretibial dermopathy.

Graves' disease affects 1–2% of females. The female:male ratio is 5:1. There is a strong association with HLA-DR3 in Caucasian people and with HLA-Bw35 and HLA-Bw46 in Asian people.

Insulin-dependent (type I) diabetes mellitus

This disorder occurs due to destruction of the insulin-producing β cells of the islets of Langerhans of the pancreas. One in 300 people in Europe and the

Systemic autoimmune diseases			
Disease	**Autoantigen**	**Diagnostic tests**	**Features**
Sjogren's syndrome	Exocrine glands	Anti-Ro and La	Reduced lacrimal and salivary gland secretion, causing dry eyes and mouth
Myositis	Muscle	ANA (Jo-1)	Muscle weakness and atrophy; mild arthritis and rashes are common
Systemic sclerosis	Nucleoli	ANA (tropoisomerase 1 and centromere)	Increased collagen deposition in skin; usually runs indolent course, but eventual involvement of internal organs occurs in most patients
Mixed connective tissue disease (MCTD)		ANA (RNP)	Features of SLE, RA, scleroderma and polymyositis; may not be a distinct entity

Fig. 2.18 Other autoimmune diseases of connective tissues. ANA, anti-nuclear antigen; RA, rheumatoid arthritis; RNP, ribonucleoprotein; SLE, systemic lupus erythematosus.

Autoimmune vasculidities		
Disease	**Diagnostic test**	**Features**
Polyarteritis nodosa	p-ANCA (myeloperoxidase)	Necrotizing inflammation of medium sized arteries. Any organ or tissue can be affected
Wegener's granulomatosis	c-ANCA (proteinase 3)	Presents with respiratory tract lesions, typically in the lungs and nose, in association with glomerulonephritis

Fig. 2.19 Autoimmune vasculidities. Antineutrophil cytoplasmic antibodies (ANCA) are specific antibodies against neutrophils. p-ANCA reacts with neutrophil myeloperoxidase and gives a perinuclear pattern on immunofluorescence; c-ANCA reacts with proteinase 3 in the cytoplasm and gives a diffuse cytoplasmic pattern in immunofluorescence.

USA are affected. An autoimmune aetiology is suspected. Over 90% of patients with the disease carry either HLA-DR3 or HLA-DR4 or both.

Immune deficiency

Immune deficiency predisposes individuals to infections, from opportunistic pathogens (those that do not normally cause disease) as well as normal pathogens. Although the cause of the deficiency can be primary or secondary, the part of the immune system that is deficient will determine the sort of infection that the individual is predisposed to. Antibody deficits result in extracellular bacterial

infection. T cell deficiencies can result in viral, fungal and intracellular bacterial infections.

Primary immune deficiencies

Primary immunodeficiencies are intrinsic, usually inherited, defects of the immune system. Different components of the immune system can be affected, including:

- Antibodies (Fig. 2.21)
- T cells (Fig. 2.22)
- Phagocytes (Fig. 2.23)
- Complement (Fig. 2.24).

It is important to recognize primary immunodeficiencies. Patients with an antibody

Fig. 2.20 Summary of organ-/cell-specific autoimmune (AI) diseases. The organ-specific autoantibodies are caused by similar genes, usually in the HLA complex. Family members therefore tend to have different organ-specific diseases. TSH, thyroid stimulating hormone.

Summary of organ/cell specific autoimmune diseases		
Disease	**Autoantigen**	**Features**
Myasthenia gravis	Acetylcholine receptor	Muscle weakness and fatiguability due to impaired neuromuscular transmission; 70% of patients have thymic hyperplasia, 10% have thymic tumour
Goodpasture's syndrome	Type IV collagen in the basement membrane of kidney and lung	Pulmonary haemorrhage and acute glomerulonephritis; peak incidence in men in their mid-20s
Pernicious anaemia	Intrinsic factor	See p. 88
AI haemolytic anaemia	Erythrocyte membrane antigens	See p. 95
AI thrombocytopenia	Platelet glycoproteins	See p. 117
Hashimoto's thyroiditis	Thyroid peroxidase	See p. 53
Graves' disease	TSH receptor	See p. 53
Type I diabetes mellitus	Islet cell antigens	See below
Coeliac disease	Tissue transglutaminase	Malabsorption due to villous atrophy in the small bowel. Diarrhoea and anaemia are common. Patients can present at any age. Treated with a gluten-free diet

Fig. 2.21 Primary antibody deficiencies. Pyogenic infections are common due to infections with encapsulated bacteria such as streptococci and staphylococci (not selective IgA deficiency).

Primary antibody deficiencies	
Disorder	**Features**
Transient physiological agammaglobulinaemia of the neonate	See Fig. 2.25
X-linked agammaglobulinaemia of Bruton	X-linked recessive disorder with defective B cell maturation. Low serum immunoglobulin levels result in recurrent pyogenic infections (seen at about 6 months). Treatment is with pooled immunoglobulin
Common variable hypogammaglobulinaemia	Heterogeneous group of disorders with normal lymphocyte numbers but abnormal B cell function; late onset (15–35 years) presenting with recurrent pyogenic infections. Treatment is with pooled immunoglobulin
Selective IgA deficiency	Occurs in 1 in 700 Caucasians but is rare in other ethnic groups; can be asymptomatic or produce recurrent infections of the respiratory and gastrointestinal tracts

Primary lymphocyte deficiencies	
Disorder	**Features**
di George syndrome (thymic hypoplasia)	Intrauterine damage to 3rd and 4th pharyngeal pouches results in failure of development of the thyroid and parathyroid glands. This results in a decrease in the number and function of T cells. Clinical features include abnormal facies, cardiac defects, hypoparathyroidism and recurrent infections
Severe combined immunodeficiency disease (SCID)	Lymphocyte deficiency and failure of thymic development due to inherited abnormalities. **X-linked SCID** is due to defects in the γ-chain of IL-2 receptor. The γ-chain forms part of several cytokine receptors including IL-7, which is needed for T cell maturation. **Autosomal recessive SCID** is caused by defects in adenosine deaminase (ADA) or purine nucleoside phosphorylase in more than 50% of cases. Both are involved in purine degradation and deficiency results in accumulation of toxic metabolites and inhibition of DNA synthesis. In both types of SCID, treatment should be by bone marrow transplant, usually before the age of two. Gene therapy might be used in the future, following success in trials that inserted the ADA gene using a retroviral vector
Wiskott–Aldrich syndrome	X-linked recessive condition characterized by normal serum IgG, low IgM and high IgA and IgE. Defective T cell function is seen, which worsens as the patient ages. Patients tend to get recurrent infections, eczema and thrombocytopenia

Fig. 2.22 Primary lymphocyte deficiencies, e.g. infections with opportunistic infections such as *Pneumocystis carinii*. T cell deficiency can cause an antibody deficiency due to lack of T-helper-cell activation of B cells.

Primary phagocyte deficiencies	
Disorder	**Features**
Neutropenia	See p. 112
Leucocyte adhesion deficiency	Lack of β$_2$-integrin molecules results in impaired adhesion and extravasation of phagocytes
Chronic granulomatous disease	Most commonly X linked (can be autosomal recessive) inheritance. Lack of NADPH oxidase (see p. 10) impairs killing of ingested pathogens, which therefore persist. Can be tested by impaired reduction of nitroblue tetrazolium by stimulated neutrophils

Fig. 2.23 Primary phagocyte deficiencies. NADPH, nicotinamide adenine dinucleotide phosphate.

deficiency will develop irreversible lung infections (bronchiectasis) unless given immunoglobulin. Children with T cell defects can be killed by infections resulting from live vaccines such as BCG.

Primary immunodeficiencies are not always pathological. Neonates do not possess a fully developed immune system at birth. In the neonatal period, infants are normally protected by maternal IgG that crossed the placenta in utero, but this is metabolized during the first months of life. Infants normally begin production of their own IgG by 3 months (Fig. 2.25). In some individuals, IgG production might not start for up to 3 years, possibly due to lack of help from T cells.

Fig. 2.24 Primary complement deficiencies. Deficiencies of almost all complement components have been described.

Primary complement deficiencies	
Disorder	**Features**
Deficiency of classical pathway components	Tend to develop immune complex disease
C3 deficiency	Prone to recurrent pyogenic infections
Deficiency of C5, C6, C7, C8, factor D, properdin	Increased susceptibility to *Neisseria* infections
C1 inhibitor deficiency	Causes hereditary angioedema

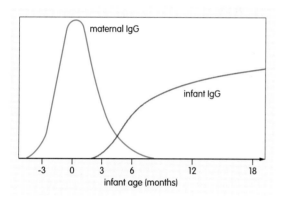

Fig. 2.25 Plasma levels of maternal and neonatal immunoglobulin in the normal-term infant. In the first 6 months of life there is a trough in immunoglobulin levels that makes infants prone to infection. IgA in breast milk can compensate. Babies born prematurely are deprived of maternal IgG and suffer exaggerated neonatal antibody deficiency.

Secondary immune deficiencies
Malnutrition and disease
Lack of dietary protein and certain elements (e.g. zinc) predisposes to secondary immunodeficiency. Infections such as malaria and measles also result in immunodeficiency.

Malignancy
Secondary immunodeficiency is particularly common with tumours that arise from the immune system, such as myeloma, lymphoma and leukaemia (see Chapter 5). Many other tumours are immunosuppressive. This is likely to provide the tumour cells with a selective advantage, because they evade destruction by cytotoxic cells.

Steroids, other drugs and radiation
Iatrogenic causes of immunosuppression are common. Immunosuppressive drugs can be given to suppress inflammatory or autoimmune disease, or to prevent rejection of transplanted material (see p. 62). Radiation and cytotoxic drugs can be used to treat malignancies and frequently cause immunosuppression.

Acquired immunodeficiency syndrome (AIDS)
Human immunodeficiency virus (HIV), a retrovirus, is the causative organism of AIDS. In 2002, the worldwide prevalence of HIV infection was over 50 million people and 5 million people died from AIDS. There are two types:
1. HIV-1: has a worldwide distribution. The structure of HIV-1 is shown in Fig. 2.26
2. HIV-2: is confined mainly to West Africa. HIV-2 has lower transmission rate than HIV-1 and runs a more benign clinical course.

Both viruses mutate rapidly, so that an infected person can contain several different strains. Transmission of the virus takes place via three routes:
1. Mucosal, i.e. by sexual contact: this is associated with other sexually transmitted diseases
2. Vertical: from mother to child (during the birth process and in breast milk, rarely transplacentally)
3. Exposure to infected blood: intravenous drug abusers, blood transfusions, needlestick injuries (0.3% risk from single exposure).

The primary infection is often asymptomatic but is marked by a flu-like illness (fever, macular rash, mouth ulcers, splenomegaly and diarrhoea) in 15% of individuals. This is followed by an asymptomatic period (median 8–10 years). It was previously thought that HIV became latent during this period. However, it is now established that HIV replication rates during this phase of the infection are very high in the lymph nodes, resulting in the production of billions of viral particles per day. The immune system is capable of containing the infection during this phase and the viral load (amount of HIV RNA in blood) in plasma remains low. Towards the end of the asymptomatic phase individuals often develop persistent generalized lymphadenopathy. The final phase of the disease is AIDS, which is characterized by:

- A low CD4 count (less than 200 cells/µl)
- Opportunistic infections such as pneumonia due to *Pneumocystis carinii*, cryptococcosis and cytomegalovirus infection
- Neoplasia, in particular Kaposi's sarcoma (caused by herpes virus 8) and B cell lymphoma
- Neurological manifestations (due to the virus itself and as a result of opportunistic infection such as cerebral toxoplasmosis).

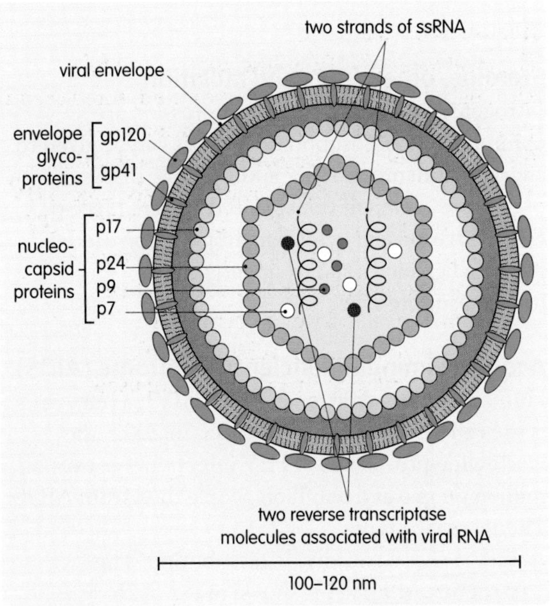

Viral load and CD4 count vary throughout HIV infection; this is illustrated in Fig. 2.27. The clinical features of AIDS relate to the CD4 count (Fig. 2.28).

Immunology of HIV infection
The gp120 antigen of HIV-1 binds the CD4 molecule on T helper (Th) cells, cells of the monocyte/macrophage lineage, and dendritic cells; gp41 is then required to enter the cell. Accessory receptors on immune cells, particularly the chemokine receptors CCR5 and CCR4, are also important. Infected monocytes, macrophages and follicular dendritic cells in lymph nodes are thought to be the major reservoir for HIV. The following changes occur:
- Depletion of peripheral blood CD4⁺ T cells
- Defects in T cell function are seen on both in vivo (failure to respond to recall antigens) and in vitro testing
- Polyclonal B cell activation occurs, resulting in hypergammaglobulinaemia

Fig. 2.26 Structure of HIV-1. The envelope glycoproteins gp120 and gp41 are hypervariable. gp120 binds CD4, allowing entry of the virus into the cell. The viral envelope is a lipid bilayer containing both viral glycoprotein antigens and host proteins.

Fig. 2.27 Variation in CD4 count and viral load during the course of HIV infection.

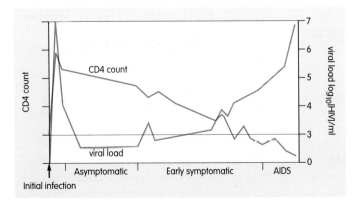

- Neutralizing antibodies directed against the gp120 and gp41 antigens are generated but do not prevent disease progression because of the high mutation rate of the virus
- Cytotoxic T cells can prevent infection (rarely) or slow progression.

Detection of HIV infection

Screening for HIV infection is performed using ELISAs to detect anti-HIV antibodies. If the ELISA is positive, confirmatory tests must be carried out, e.g. a Western blot, which detects antibodies against specific HIV proteins. Seroconversion (production of antibodies) might not take place until 3 months after infection, hence there is a window period when ELISA will be negative. This is a potential problem in blood transfusion (see p. 144).

In infants, anti-HIV IgG can be maternally derived and persist for up to 18 months, making diagnosis of HIV by ELISA unreliable. Detection of HIV by polymerase chain reaction (PCR) is used to confirm HIV infection in neonates.

Treatment of HIV

The treatment of HIV is now very successful. Although the infection cannot be cured, survival and quality of life have been profoundly increased. Treatment is with antiretrovirals and antibiotics:

- **Antiretroviral therapy:** antiretrovirals target HIV at various points of its lifecycle (Fig. 2.29). HIV mutates rapidly and can become resistant to drugs. This is less likely to happen when combinations of different classes of antiretrovirals, known as highly active antiretroviral therapy (HAART) are used.

Clinical infections at different CD4 counts	
CD4 count	Infection
<400	Tuberculosis
<300	Kaposi's sarcoma Oesophageal candidiasis
<200	Pneumocystis carinii pneumonia (PCP) Toxoplasmosis
<100	Mycobacterium avium intracellulare CMV retinitis

Fig. 2.28 Clinical infections at different CD4 counts. CMV, cytomegalovirus.

Fig. 2.29 Antiretroviral agents in current use and their site of action in the lifecycle of HIV. AZT, azidothymidine.

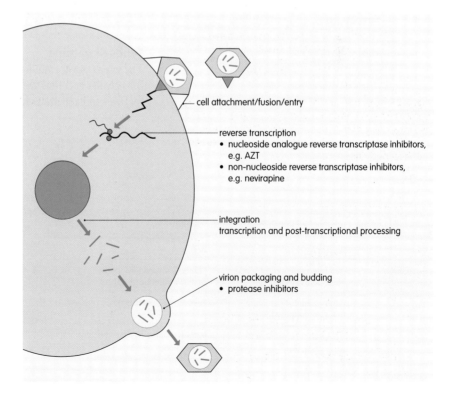

cell attachment/fusion/entry

reverse transcription
- nucleoside analogue reverse transcriptase inhibitors, e.g. AZT
- non-nucleoside reverse transcriptase inhibitors, e.g. nevirapine

integration
transcription and post-transcriptional processing

virion packaging and budding
- protease inhibitors

HAART is usually initiated when viral load rises late in infection. It usually results in a reduction of viral load to undetectable levels and an increase in CD4 counts, with concomitant restoration of immune competence

- **Antibiotic prophylaxis and treatment of infection:** prophylaxis against infections such as *Pneumocystis carinii* and *Toxoplasma gondii* is effective and usually given when the CD4 count is less than 200/μl. It has been shown that antibiotic prophylaxis can be safely stopped following immune restoration using treatment with HAART.

Immunization

Concepts of immunization

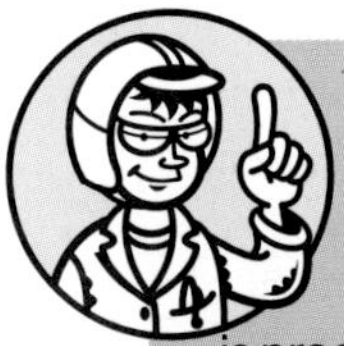

It is important to be able to explain the difference between active and passive immunity. Active immunity is produced by the body in response to antigen (either infection or vaccination). In vaccination, active immunity produces a response to antigen that is given to the patient. Preformed antibodies are used in passive immunization.

Immunity can be achieved by passive or active immunization (Fig. 2.30).

Active immunization

Active immunization results from contact with antigens, either through natural infection or by vaccination. Individuals exhibit a primary immune response, with clonal expansion of B and T cells and formation of memory cells. Subsequent exposure to the same antigen will induce a secondary immune response (see p. 7).

Vaccination

Vaccination is a form of active immunization that induces specific immunity to a particular pathogen. The aim is to produce a rapid, protective immune response on re-exposure to that pathogen. An ideal vaccine is:

- Safe, with minimal side-effects and free from contaminating substances
- Immunogenic, activating the required branches of the immune system, inducing long-lasting local and systemic immunity
- Heat stable, because there are difficulties with refrigeration, particularly in tropical countries
- Inexpensive, an important consideration, especially in developing countries.

Types of vaccine

The types of vaccine in current use are listed in Fig. 2.31. Most vaccines are live attenuated or killed; the features of each are compared in Fig. 2.32. The

Comparison of passive and active immunity		
	Passive	**Active**
Features	Preformed immunoglobulins transferred to individual	Contact with antigen induces adaptive immune response
	Large amounts of antibody available immediately	Takes some time to develop immunity
	Short lifespan of antibodies	Long-lived immunity induced
Examples	Antitetanus toxin antibody	Natural exposure; vaccination

Fig. 2.30 Comparison of passive and active immunity.

Different types of vaccine

Vaccine	Features	Examples
Live attenuated	Attenuation achieved by repeated culture on artificial media or by serial passage in animals; immunogenicity is retained, but virulence is significantly diminished	Oral polio (Sabin), BCG, rubella, measles, mumps
Killed	Intact organisms killed by exposure to heat or chemicals, e.g. formalin	Intramuscular polio (Salk), pertussis
Subunit	Purified, protective immunity-inducing antigenic components; often surface antigens	Influenza, pneumococccal
Recombinant	Genes encoding epitopes, which elicit protective immunity, are inserted into pro- or eukaryotic cells; large quantities of vaccine are produced rapidly	Hepatitis B surface antigen (produced in yeast cells)
Toxoids	Bacterial toxins inactivated by heat or chemicals	Diphtheria, tetanus
Conjugates	Polysaccharide antigen is linked to protein carrier to enhance immunogenicity	*Haemophilus influenzae* type B (Hib), meningococcal

Fig. 2.31 Different types of vaccine in use in the UK today. BCG, Bacille Calmette–Guèrin.

Features of live versus killed vaccines

Feature	Live attenuated vaccine	Killed vaccine
Level of immunity induced	High: organism replicates (mimicking natural infection)	Low: non-replicating organisms produce a short-lived stimulus
Cell-mediated response	Good: antigens are processed and presented with MHC molecules	Poor
Local immunity	Good	Poor
Cost	Expensive to produce and administer	Cheaper than live vaccines
Reversion to virulence	Possible but rare	No (therefore safe for immunocompromised and pregnant patients)
Stability	Heat labile	Heat stable
Risk of contamination	Possible, e.g. by virus in cell media	N/a

Fig. 2.32 Features of live versus killed vaccines. The genes of attenuated organisms can differ from the wild type by just a few base pairs. It is relatively easy for them to mutate back to the disease-causing strain. MHC, major histocompatibility complex; N/a, not applicable.

routine immunization schedule used in the UK is shown in Fig. 2.33.

Vaccines are not 100% efficacious. A small proportion of individuals receiving vaccination will not respond adequately. However, by immunizing the majority of the population, non-responders are unlikely to come into contact with the virus because the viral reservoir is reduced (herd immunity).

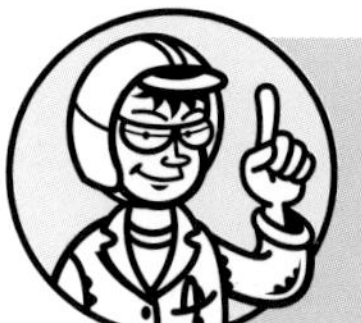

It is possible to enhance the immune response to vaccines by using adjuvants. Adjuvants, e.g. aluminium salts and Bordetella pertussis, are non-specific.

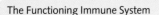

UK immunization schedule	
Age	**Vaccine**
Neonate (certain groups)	BCG, Hep B
2, 3, 4 months	Diphtheria/tetanus/pertussis Oral polio Hib Meningococcus C
12–15 months	MMR
4–5 years	MMR, diphtheria, tetanus, acellular pertussis
10–14 years	BCG
13–18 years	Boosters for diphtheria, tetanus, oral polio
Adult	Boosters for tetanus and polio Occupational or lifestyle risk
65 years	Influenza
Any age	Influenza, pneumococcus Occupation Hep A, Hep B Travel, e.g. Yellow fever

Fig. 2.33 Routine immunization schedule used in the UK. BCG, Bacille Calmette–Guérin; Hep, hepatitis; Hib, *Haemophilus influenzae* type B; MMR, measles, mumps, rubella.

Passive immunization

Passive immunization involves the transfer of preformed immunoglobulins to an individual. Contact with antigen is not required. Passive immunization is used if an individual is exposed to an organism to which he or she does not have active immunity. Passive immunization can be used to:
- Prevent Hepatitis A and B infection
- Prevent varicella zoster
- Treat snake bites (anti-venom).

Transplantation

Mechanisms of solid organ transplant rejection

Autologous grafts are grafts moved from one part of the body to another, e.g. skin grafts.
Syngeneic grafts are between genetically identical individuals, e.g. monozygotic twins.
Allogeneic grafts are between individuals of the same species.
Xenogeneic grafts are between different species.

Unless the donor and recipient are immunologically identical, the recipient will mount a rejection response against 'foreign' antigens expressed by the graft. The most important graft antigens responsible for an immune response in the recipient are the MHC molecules (see p. 17). However, even when the donor and recipient are genetically identical at the MHC loci, graft rejection can occur due to differences at other loci, which encode minor histocompatibility antigens. A rejection response can lead to loss of a graft. There are three types of graft rejection (Fig. 2.34):
1. Hyperacute
2. Acute cellular
3. Chronic.

Strategies for preventing rejection
HLA typing and antibody cross-matching
The ideal match is that between monozygotic twins. In all other situations there will be some genetic disparity between donor and recipient. The aim of matching is to minimize genetic differences between donor and recipient. Both the donor and recipient will by HLA typed.

Antirejection therapy
Immunosuppressive drugs can be used to prevent rejection by suppressing antibody and T cell responses. Examples of drugs used include:

Fig. 2.34 Patterns of graft rejection. HLA, human leucocyte antigen.

Patterns of graft rejection		
Type	**Mechanism**	**Prevention**
Hyperacute (minutes–hours)	Pre-existing antidonor antibodies	Perform cross-match of donor cells and recipient's serum, check for ABO compatibility
Acute cellular (days–weeks)	T cell mediated	HLA matching of donor and recipient, antirejection therapy
Chronic (months–years)	Unclear	HLA matching

Fig. 2.35 Common transplants.

Common transplants	
Transplant	**Notes**
Kidney	Live or cadaveric donor; the fewer the MHC mismatches, the greater the success rate; must be ABO compatible
Heart	Matching is beneficial, but often time is a more pressing concern
Liver	No evidence to suggest that matching affects graft survival; rejection less aggressive than for other organs
Skin graft	Most grafts are autologous, but allografts can be used to protect burns patients
Corneal graft	Matching (class II MHC) is required only if a previous graft was vascularized
Stem cell	Host-versus-graft (HVG) or graft-versus-host (GVH) responses possible. The transplant must be well matched and antirejection therapy used. Host immune cells are destroyed by irradiation prior to transplant (avoids HVG). T cells are depleted from the graft (avoids GVH) using monoclonal antibody and complement

- Steroids: these are anti-inflammatory (see p. 45)
- Azathioprine: an antiproliferative drug
- Tacrolimus and ciclosporin: inhibit signalling in T cells.

The disadvantage of such non-specific therapy is that the recipient is at increased risk of opportunistic infections (e.g. cytomegalovirus) and certain malignancies. Newer, more selective agents are being developed, including anti-CD3 monoclonal antibodies.

Common types of transplantation performed today are summarized in Fig. 2.35.

Stem cell transplant

Stem cell transplants are used in the treatment of some cancers and primary immunodeficiencies. Stem cells are obtained from bone marrow or blood. Imperfectly matched stem cells can be rejected by the recipient. In addition, stem cells give rise to lymphocytes, which can attack the host causing acute or chronic graft-versus-host disease.

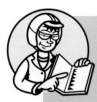

- Describe the processes that occur for neutrophils to extravasate at sites of inflammation.
- Which chemicals mediate acute inflammation?
- What are the consequences of acute and chronic inflammation?
- Outline the immune responses to viruses, bacteria and protozoa.
- What mechanisms do pathogens use to evade the immune response?
- What is hypersensitivity and how is it classified?
- What immune mechanisms result in hypersensitivity?
- What drugs are used to reduce inflammation, and how do they act?
- Explain how ELISA could be used to diagnose the presence of an antigen in serum.
- Give examples of common allergic conditions and the allergens that cause them.
- How does the body prevent self-reactive lymphocytes from causing autoimmune disease?
- What role do infection and human leucocyte antigen (HLA) molecules play in autoimmunity?
- What pathological processes occur in rheumatoid arthritis?
- What are the causes and features of primary immunodeficiency?
- What are the causes of secondary immunodeficiencies?
- Describe the immunology, laboratory features and diagnosis of HIV infection.
- What are the differences between active and passive immunity?
- What is the routine immunization schedule in the UK?
- Compare and contrast live and killed vaccines.
- Why are transplanted organs rejected and what steps are taken to prevent this?

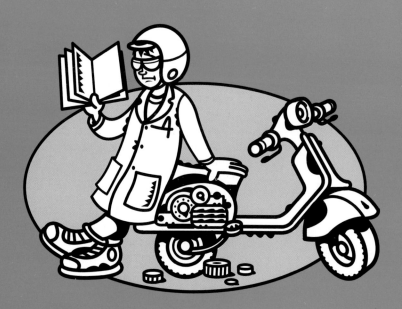

HAEMATOLOGY

3. Principles of Haematology

The second part of this book covers haematology, and is organized around the various cell types. The production of blood cells, bone marrow and the function of the spleen are discussed in this chapter. Chapter 4 looks more closely at oxygen transport and the clinical importance of red blood cells. This is followed by the function and clinical relevance of white blood cells. The last three chapters explore haemostasis, including platelets, important haematological investigations and blood transfusion.

Overview of haematology—the cell lines

All blood cells are derived from a common or 'pluripotent' stem cell, a process known as haemopoiesis. The stem cell produces lineage-committed progenitors that develop into the cells seen in blood. Each haemopoietic cell type has an important physiological role.

Red blood cells:

- **Erythrocytes:** utilize haemoglobin to transport oxygen and carbon dioxide between the lungs and the rest of the body (see Chapter 4).

White blood cells (for immune functions see Chapter 1; for cytological appearance see Chapter 5):

- **Neutrophils:** phagocytose foreign material or dead/damaged cells at sites of inflammation and activate bactericidal mechanisms
- **Eosinophils:** important in the host defence against parasites (coated in antibody). They are also involved in allergic responses
- **Basophils:** become mast cells in tissues where they are coated with IgE and release histamine
- **Monocytes:** enter tissues to become macrophages. Monocyte-derived cells are found throughout the body as part of the reticuloendothelial system. They phagocytose pathogens and cellular debris and produce various cytokines. They also process and present antigen to lymphocytes as part of the adaptive immune response

- **B lymphocytes:** as plasma cells they are responsible for immunoglobulin production. They can also become memory B cells
- **T lymphocytes:** cytotoxic $CD8^+$ T cells kill cells infected by intracellular organisms. $CD4^+$ T helper cells produce cytokines to activate B cells or macrophages
- **Natural killer (NK) cells:** kill cells they detect as foreign either directly or via antibody-dependent cell-mediated cytotoxicity
- **Platelets:** megakaryocyte fragments involved in the haemostatic response to vascular injury (coagulation). (see Chapter 6).

Haemopoiesis and its regulation

Haemopoiesis is the formation and development of blood cells. This process depends upon stem cells, which divide to leave both a reserve population and cells committed to differentiating into the various blood cell lines (Fig. 3.1). Differentiation occurs along one of three lineages:

1. Erythroid → erythrocytes
2. Lymphoid → B and T lymphocytes and NK cells
3. Myeloid → neutrophils, basophils, eosinophils, monocytes and megakaryocytes.

Sites of haemopoiesis
The main site of haemopoiesis changes during fetal development and maturation:
- Conception to 6 weeks: fetal yolk sac
- 6 weeks to 6 months: fetal liver and spleen
- 6 months onwards: bone marrow.

Progenitor cells
In vitro, haemopoietic progenitors are detected via assays that identify cells capable of producing colonies (a colony-forming unit or CFU). Granulocytes, erythrocytes, monocytes and megakaryocytes are produced from a precursor known as CFU-GEMM. This divides into an erythroid progenitor (CFU-E), a megakaryocyte precursor, an eosinophil precursor and a

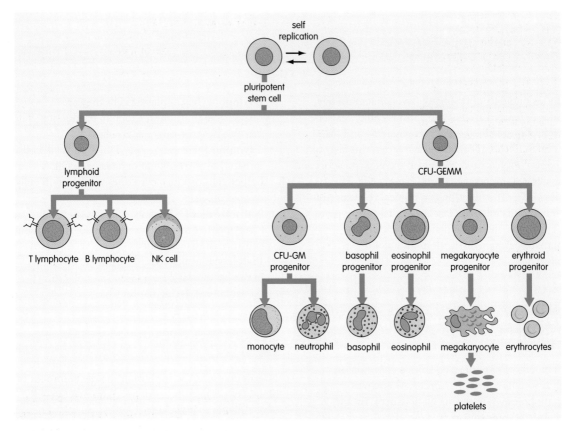

Fig. 3.1 Overview of haemopoiesis. Blood cells are derived from pluripotent stem cells usually found in the bone marrow. Exposure to different growth factors promotes the development of the different cell lines. CFU-GEMM, granulocyte, erythrocyte, monocyte, megakaryocyte colony-forming unit; CFU-GM, granulocyte, monocyte colony-forming unit; NK, natural killer.

granulocyte/monocyte precursor (CFU-GM). Lymphoid precursors become B cells or NK cells in the bone marrow or travel to the thymus where they develop into T cells.

Growth factors

Cytokines and other growth factors regulate haemopoiesis (Fig. 3.2). These factors are glycoproteins produced in the bone marrow, liver and kidneys. Binding of the growth factor to surface receptors can trigger replication, differentiation or functional activation, or they can inhibit apoptosis. Following stimulation by interferon-1 or tumour necrosis factor (TNF), stromal cells in the bone marrow produce many growth factors. Several growth factors, known as colony stimulating factors (CSFs), have been identified:

- Multilineage CSF (IL-3): acts early in haemopoiesis to induce non-lymphoid cell production
- Granulocyte–macrophage CSF: acts later on the same cells
- Macrophage CSF and granulocyte CSF: are involved later still to produce monocytes and neutrophils.

Clinical use of growth factors

Erythropoietin replacement is given to patients in renal failure to prevent anaemia. Other CSFs such as G-CSF, GM-CSF and thrombopoietin are also in use—most commonly with chemotherapy regimes or where bone marrow eradication or harvesting is to take place.

Fig. 3.2 Growth factors in haemopoiesis. CFU-GEMM, granulocyte, erythrocyte, monocyte, megakaryocyte colony-forming unit; CFU-GM, granulocyte, monocyte colony-forming unit; GM-CSF, granulocyte–macrophage colony-stimulating factor; IL, interleukin; M-CSF, macrophage colony-stimulating factor, TNF tumour necrosis factor.

Haemopoietic growth factors	
Factor	**Site of action**
Stem cell factor	Pluripotent cells
IL-3	CFU-GEMM
GM-CSF	CFU-GM
G-CSF	Granulocyte precursor
M-CSF	Monocyte precursor
IL-5	Eosinophil progenitors
Erythropoietin	Erythrocyte progenitors
Thrombopoietin	Megakaryocyte progenitors
IL-6	B cell precursors
IL-2	T cell precursors
IL-1 and TNF	Stromal cells

Bone marrow

Haemopoiesis occurs in the entire skeleton of the newborn, but haemopoietic tissue is restricted to the central skeleton (sternum, vertebrae, ribs, hip bones, clavicles and cranial bones) and the proximal ends of long bones in the adult.

Bone marrow is classified as red (approximately 50% of red marrow is haemopoietic) or yellow (composed mostly of fat, no longer productive of blood cells). If the requirement for blood cells is very large, the small population of precursor cells in yellow marrow can be reactivated. In addition, the liver and spleen can resume their fetal haemopoietic role.

Structure

The red marrow provides a suitable microenvironment for stem cell growth and development. It has two main components:

1. Specialized fibroblasts, known as adventitial reticular cells, which secrete a framework of reticulin fibres (fine collagen fibres), forming a meshwork that is essential to support developing blood cells
2. A network of blood sinusoids, lined by a single layer of endothelial cells, which interconnect via

tight junctions. The vascular sinuses support the haemopoietic cells. They drain into a large central sinus that channels the blood into the systemic venous circulation. The endothelium of the sinusoids exhibits transient cytoplasmic pores, which allow passage of newly formed cells into the circulation.

Haemopoiesis takes place in haemopoietic cords or islands located between the vascular sinuses (Fig. 3.3). Macrophages found within the haemopoietic cords at the centre of each focal group contain stored iron in the form of ferritin and haemosiderin. They have three main functions:

1. Transfer of iron to developing erythroblasts for haemoglobin synthesis
2. Phagocytosis of the cellular debris of haemopoiesis
3. Regulation of haemopoietic cell differentiation and maturation.

Generation of B cells

Bone marrow is considered to be a primary lymphoid organ, i.e. it generates lymphocytes. B-cell development is dependent on stromal cells in the bone marrow. The stroma forms specific adhesion contacts with pro-B cells. As B cells develop they

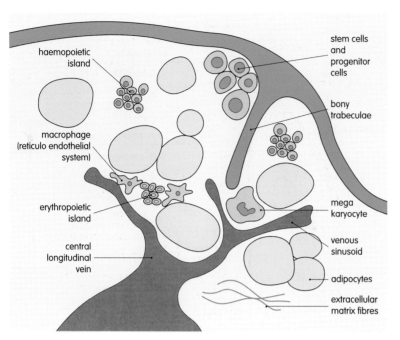

Fig. 3.3 Bone marrow structure. Haemopoietic islands of developing blood cells are interspersed between bony trabeculae and fat cells. A connective tissue stroma of reticular cells and fibres support the developing cells. Venous plexuses, draining into a central longitudinal vein, transport developed cells out of the bone marrow.

migrate towards the central axis of the marrow cavity and become less dependent on stromal contact. Immature B cells that bind to self cell-surface antigen are removed from the repertoire at this stage. B cells move to the spleen or lymph nodes for final maturation. T lymphocyte precursors leave the bone marrow early in development and are transferred to the thymus for maturation.

The spleen

The spleen is a secondary lymphoid organ. It is the site of B and T cell proliferation and of antibody formation, and an important component of the reticuloendothelial system. It is specialized to filter blood much as the lymph nodes filter lymph. Blood supply to the spleen is via the splenic artery. Blood is drained via the splenic veins, which join the superior mesenteric vein to form the portal vein.

The spleen is an intraperitoneal organ, its relations comprise:

- Anteriorly: the stomach, tail of the pancreas, and left colic flexure
- Medially: the left kidney
- Posteriorly: the diaphragm, left pleura, left lung and ribs 9–11.

Structure

The spleen is surrounded by a dense, irregular fibroelastic connective tissue capsule that projects fibres, known as trabeculae, into the organ. The two main types of tissues found within the spleen are red pulp and white pulp. These are separated by a marginal zone (Fig. 3.4).

Red pulp

The red pulp is made up of venous sinuses and splenic cords. The splenic cords are composed of reticular fibres, reticular cells, plasma cells, phagocytes and some B cells. The red pulp removes old or defective erythrocytes and platelets from the circulation.

White pulp and marginal zone

The central arteriole is surrounded by a periarteriolar lymphoid sheath (PALS), which predominantly contains T cells. These branch between B cell follicles that could be primary (unstimulated) but will be secondary (stimulated) in most patients. The PALS and follicles constitute the white pulp. The white pulp is surrounded by a marginal zone containing plasma cells, T and B lymphocytes, macrophages and dendritic cells. The marginal zone is supplied by venous sinuses that have gaps as wide

Fig. 3.4 Structure of the spleen. Arterioles entering the spleen are surrounded by T lymphocytes, the periarteriolar lymphoid sheath (PALS). Along with B cells organized into follicles, this constitutes the white pulp. These structures are surrounded by a marginal zone containing plasma cells, lymphocytes, macrophages and dendritic cells. The rest of the spleen is composed of splenic cords (red pulp) and venous sinuses.

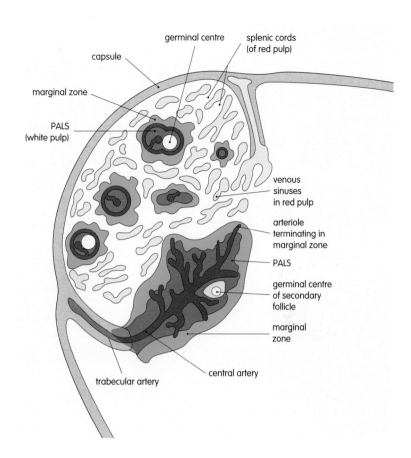

as 2–3 μm between the endothelial cells. The following functions occur in the marginal zone:

- Antigen-presenting cells sample blood for antigens
- Lymphocytes exit the circulation and migrate to their respective domains
- Monocytes enter the spleen and become macrophages. Here they can attack blood-borne microorganisms
- Lymphocytes and dendritic cells come into contact, allowing initiation of an immune response.

The spleen also acts as a reservoir for platelets, erythrocytes and granulocytes.

Embryology

The spleen begins as a mesodermal proliferation in the primitive gut during the 5th week of fetal development. It is connected to the body wall by the lienorenal ligament and to the stomach by the gastrolienal ligament.

Disorders of the spleen
Splenomegaly

Splenomegaly—enlargement of the spleen—is a frequent clinical finding that can occur in a number of different disorders (Fig. 3.5). The causes of splenomegaly are subject to geographical variation; haemolytic disorders predominate in the UK whereas parasitic causes are very common in tropical countries.

Hypersplenism

Hypersplenism can occur in any disorder where the spleen is enlarged. It is characterized by:

- Splenomegaly
- Anaemia, leucopenia and thrombocytopenia, either singly or in any combination
- Normal cellular or hypercellular bone marrow.

In the enlarged spleen there is increased sequestration of blood cells, which are lysed by macrophages. Splenectomy corrects the blood cytopenias.

Causes of splenomegaly		
Haematological		Lymphomas and leukaemias Polycythaemia rubra vera Haemolytic anaemias Haemoglobinopathies
Infectious	Acute	Infectious mononucleosis Typhoid fever Toxoplasmosis Bacterial endocarditis
	Chronic	Tuberculosis Brucellosis Syphilis Chronic bacteraemia Histoplasmosis
	Parasitic	Malaria Schistosomiasis Leishmaniasis Echinococcosis Trypanosomiasis
Portal hypertension		Liver cirrhosis Cardiac failure (right sided) Hepatic, portal, or splenic vein thrombosis
Immunological		Rheumatoid arthritis Felty's syndrome (hypersplenism in rheumatoid arthritis) Systemic lupus erythematosus Sarcoidosis
Storage diseases		Gaucher's disease Niemann–Pick disease
Others		Malignancies (rare) Cysts Amyloid Hyperthyroidism

Fig. 3.5 Causes of splenomegaly.

Congestive splenomegaly

Congestive splenomegaly is caused by persistent venous congestion. Systemic, prehepatic and hepatic causes are the most important.

Splenic infarction

Splenic infarction is relatively common and is caused by the occlusion of the splenic artery or its major branches. Emboli are the most common cause but local thrombi caused by sickle-cell disease and myeloproliferative disorders also occur. Infarcts might be single or multiple. Splenic atrophy can also occur in association with coeliac disease and dermatitis herpetiformis. These patients are at risk from certain infections.

Neoplasms of the spleen

Primary splenic neoplasms are very rare. The most common neoplasms found in the spleen are lymphomas and leukaemias. Haematogenous metastatic spread to the spleen does occur.

Congenital abnormalities

Congenital asplenia (absence of the spleen) is relatively rare and usually occurs in conjunction with other congenital abnormalities. Approximately 10% of the population have accessory spleens.

Rupture of the spleen

Causes include:

- Infections, e.g. infectious mononucleosis
- Haemopoietic disorders, e.g. myelofibrosis
- Abdominal trauma, e.g. road-traffic accidents.

Splenectomy

Indications for splenectomy (removal of the spleen) include:

- Severe splenic trauma
- Splenic cysts
- Treatment of idiopathic thrombocytopenic purpura
- Treatment of autoimmune or other types of haemolysis
- Tumours of the spleen and adjacent organs.

Following splenectomy, the patient should be encouraged to mobilize as soon as possible because they are at high risk of thrombosis. There is a lifelong increased risk of infection, particularly encapsulated organisms (e.g. *Neisseria meningitides*, *Streptococcus pneumoniae*, *Haemophilus influenzae*). The following steps should be taken:

- Pneumococcal vaccine should be given (preferably more than 2 weeks before surgery), with boosters every 5–10 years
- Hib and meningococcal vaccine should also be given
- Lifelong prophylactic antibiotics are recommended
- Standby antibiotic should be kept by the patient, to start if any symptoms of infection develop
- Patients should be warned that tropical infections (e.g. malaria) are more likely to be severe
- Urgent hospital admission if infection develops.

- Which lymphoid cells are found in the blood?
- Which blood cells are phagocytic?
- Why are some blood cells coated in antibodies?
- Describe where blood cells are generated at different stages of development?
- Which factors regulate haemopoiesis?
- How is the bone marrow specialized to produce blood cells?
- What is the important role of bone marrow macrophages in haemopoiesis?
- What is the structure of the spleen?
- Why is the marginal zone of the spleen important for the immune response?
- What are the consequences of an enlarged spleen?

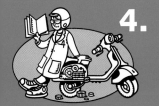

4. Red Blood Cells and Haemoglobin

Structure and function of erythrocytes

Erythrocyte structure

Erythrocytes are mature red cells with an average lifespan of 120 days (Fig. 4.1). The normal concentration of erythrocytes in the blood is 3.9–6.5 $\times 10^{12}$/L. Erythrocytes:

- Are not nucleated and contain no organelles
- Contain millions of molecules of haemoglobin, an oxygen-carrying pigment that gives blood its red colour
- Have a characteristic biconcave discoid shape on blood smears. This gives a 20–30% larger surface area than a sphere of the same volume
- Have an average diameter of 7.2 μm
- Are highly flexible and deform readily, allowing passage through vessels of the microvasculature only 3 μm in diameter.

Erythrocyte function

The primary function of erythrocytes is carriage of oxygen (O_2) and carbon dioxide (CO_2) between the lungs and tissues. The large surface area facilitates this function. They also play an important role in pH buffering.

Gas exchange and transport

The body's resting requirement for O_2 is 250 mL/min. About 200 mL of oxygen is transported in each litre of blood. Multiplied by resting cardiac output (~5 L/min), this means that 1000 mL of O_2 is transported each minute. A small amount of O_2 is dissolved in the blood but the majority is transported by haemoglobin. The oxygen content of the blood depends on three factors:

1. The concentration of haemoglobin
2. The affinity of haemoglobin for oxygen (see p. 81)
3. The solubility of oxygen in the blood (small effect).

CO_2 is carried in the blood in three forms (Fig. 4.2):

1. ~90% as bicarbonate
2. ~5% in the form of carbamino compounds (CO_2 combines with the amino groups of plasma proteins and haemoglobin)
3. ~5% in physical solution (CO_2 is over 20 times more soluble in blood than is O_2).

The large bicarbonate stores of CO_2 are an important pH buffer within the blood. CO_2 levels are tightly regulated by changes in ventilation.

Electrolyte balance

Chloride, potassium and hydrogen ions are transported across the red-cell membrane. One consequence of this is that, in blood stored for transfusion, the extracellular potassium level is quite high due to disruption of active transport. In large transfusions there is potential for hyperkalaemia in some cases.

Erythropoiesis

Erythropoiesis (Fig. 4.3) is the production of red blood cells, from the CFU-GEMM (granulocyte, erythrocyte, monocyte, megakaryocyte) progenitor.

Sequence of erythropoiesis

Erythropoiesis occurs in erythroblastic islands within the bone marrow. These contain macrophages, which supply iron to the surrounding erythroid progenitor cells. The entire sequence (from stem cell to erythrocyte) takes approximately 1 week. Maturation is characterized by the following stages:

- Pronormoblast
- Early, intermediate, and late normoblasts
- Reticulocyte
- Erythrocyte.

The production of new blood cells balances the removal of mature cells by the spleen. Following severe erythrocyte depletion, e.g. due to haemolysis, the rate of erythropoiesis in the bone marrow increases. Nucleated precursors and an increased number of reticulocytes will also appear in the peripheral blood.

Ineffective erythropoiesis

Each pronormoblast can potentially give rise to 16 erythrocytes, but some normoblasts fail to develop and are phagocytosed by bone marrow macrophages. In a healthy individual, the amount of this 'ineffective erythropoiesis' is small.

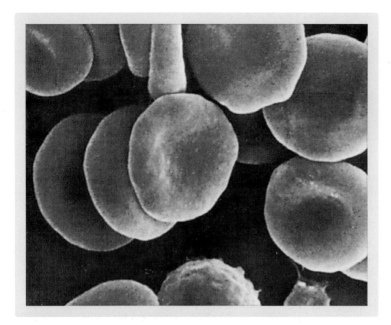

Fig. 4.1 Scanning electron micrograph of red blood cells showing their characteristic discoid, biconcave shape (courtesy Dr Trevor Gray).

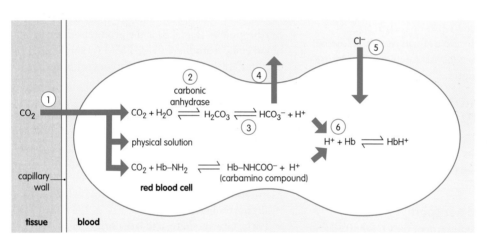

Fig. 4.2 Carbon dioxide (CO_2) transport. CO_2 is transported in both red blood cells and the plasma. Only the intracellular pathways are shown. (1) CO_2 moves along a concentration gradient from tissue to blood. (2) Carbonic anhydrase (not present in plasma) catalyses the formation of carbonic acid (H_2CO_3) from H_2O and CO_2. (3) H_2CO_3 dissociates into protons (H^+) and bicarbonate ions (HCO_3^-). (4) HCO_3^- diffuse along a concentration gradient into the plasma. (5) Chloride ions (Cl^-) enter the cell to maintain electroneutrality, a process known as the 'chloride shift'. (6) H^+, produced as a result of the dissociation of H_2CO_3 and carbamino compounds, is not able to leave the cell. Imidazole groups on the haemoglobin molecule buffer the protons.

Regulation of erythropoiesis

The principal factor regulating erythropoiesis is a hormone called erythropoietin.

Erythropoietin (EPO)

EPO is a heavily glycosylated polypeptide. It is 165 amino acids in length and weighs ~30400kDa. It is secreted by:

- Endothelial cells of the peritubular capillaries in the renal cortex (90%)
- Kupffer cells and hepatocytes in the liver (10%).

Control of erythropoietin drive

The major stimulus for secretion is hypoxia. This can be caused by any factor that gives rise to decreased oxygen transport to tissues relative to tissue demand (Fig. 4.4).

Fig. 4.3 Red cell precursors and the sequence of erythropoiesis. The appearance is that seen with the routine Romanowsky stain, unless otherwise specified.

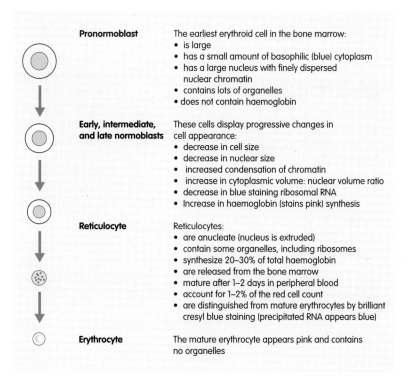

Pronormoblast

The earliest erythroid cell in the bone marrow:
• is large
• has a small amount of basophilic (blue) cytoplasm
• has a large nucleus with finely dispersed nuclear chromatin
• contains lots of organelles
• does not contain haemoglobin

Early, intermediate, and late normoblasts

These cells display progressive changes in cell appearance:
• decrease in cell size
• decrease in nuclear size
• increased condensation of chromatin
• increase in cytoplasmic volume: nuclear volume ratio
• decrease in blue staining ribosomal RNA
• Increase in haemoglobin (stains pink) synthesis

Reticulocyte

Reticulocytes:
• are anucleate (nucleus is extruded)
• contain some organelles, including ribosomes
• synthesize 20–30% of total haemoglobin
• are released from the bone marrow
• mature after 1–2 days in peripheral blood
• account for 1–2% of the red cell count
• are distinguished from mature erythrocytes by brilliant cresyl blue staining (precipitated RNA appears blue)

Erythrocyte

The mature erythrocyte appears pink and contains no organelles

Fig. 4.4 Regulation of erythropoietin (EPO) production. Reduced oxygen (O_2) supply to renal sensors stimulates EPO production. If this is chronically activated extramedullary erythropoiesis can occur.

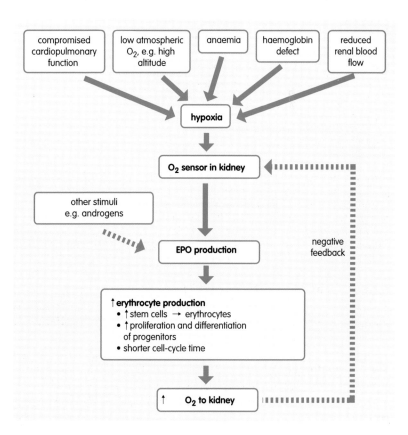

Chronic renal disease (decrease in, or a complete loss of, renal mass) or bilateral nephrectomy can lead to decreased production of EPO, resulting in anaemia. Renal cell carcinomas can produce excess EPO, resulting in an erythrocytosis.

Recombinant EPO, produced in animal cells, is currently used for:

- Anaemia due to renal failure
- Autologous blood transfusions
- After chemotherapy or bone marrow transplantation
- Anaemia of chronic disease.

Erythropoiesis is also regulated by the availability of red cell components, most importantly iron, folic acid, and vitamin B_{12}.

Iron and haem metabolism

Iron metabolism
Uptake and excretion of iron
Normal uptake and excretion of iron is illustrated in Fig. 4.5. The total iron store of the body is around 4g, mainly as haemoglobin (Fig. 4.6). The daily requirement is normally around 1 mg. Absorption is controlled by proteins in the gut. The rate of iron transfer from epithelial cells to plasma responds to iron requirements, e.g. it is high when stores are low or the rate of erythropoiesis is high.

Iron transport proteins
Free iron is toxic and is therefore incorporated into haem or bound to protein within the body.

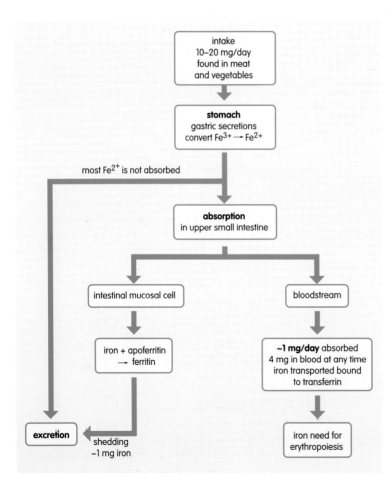

Fig. 4.5 Uptake and excretion of iron. Iron is converted in the stomach from Fe^{3+} to Fe^{2+}. This process is promoted by ascorbic acid and other reducing agents and inhibited by phytates, tannic acid and tetracycline. The ferrous form, Fe^{2+}, is actively absorbed in the duodenum and jejunum. Within intestinal mucosal cells, some iron binds apoferritin to form ferritin, a storage compound. The rest is transported, by transferrin in the blood, to storage compartments and the bone marrow. A total of 1mg of iron is absorbed into the bloodstream each day. Total daily iron turnover is ~25mg. Iron in shed mucosal cells or not absorbed from the diet is excreted in the faeces, although a small amount is lost from shed skin cells and in the urine. Extra iron is lost during menstruation (1.5mg solidus day compared with 1mg normally).

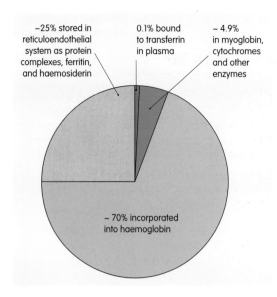

Fig. 4.6 Distribution of iron in the body.

Transferrin transports up to two molecules of iron to tissues that have transferrin receptors, e.g. bone marrow. Ferritin is a water-soluble compound, consisting of protein and iron. Haemosiderin is insoluble and consists of aggregates of ferritin that have partially lost their protein component.

Iron overload

There is no mechanism for the excretion of excess iron. Consequently, iron overload can occur as a result of:

- Increased absorption
- Parenteral administration.

Increased absorption

This can be either primary or secondary, and results from the following:

- Primary/hereditary haemochromatosis—an autosomal recessive disorder characterized by excessive intestinal absorption of iron
- Erythroid hyperplasia secondary to ineffective erythropoiesis or haemolysis, e.g. thalassaemia syndromes
- Dietary excess (rare)
- Inappropriate oral therapy.

Parenteral administration

- Multiple blood transfusions (1 unit of blood contains ~250mg of iron)
- Inappropriate parenteral iron therapy.

Treatment

It is important to start therapy as soon as possible to prevent irreversible organ damage. Options include:

- Dietary advice (decrease intake of iron, increase intake of natural chelators)
- Venesection
- Chelation therapy—desferrioxamine is an iron-chelating agent that is administered subcutaneously.

The clinical symptoms of iron overload are due to iron deposition. They include:
- Cardiomyopathy → dysrhythmias and heart failure.
- Reduction in growth and sexual development in children.
- Reduced pituitary, thyroid and parathyroid function.
- Diabetes mellitus.
- Cirrhosis and haemosiderosis of the liver.
- Excessive melanin skin pigmentation.

Haem metabolism

Haem belongs to a family of compounds known as the porphyrins, which are characterized by the presence of a tetrapyrrole ring. Haem is an iron-containing derivative, the iron atom being located at the centre of the tetrapyrrole ring of protoporphyrin IX. The haem group is responsible for the oxygen-binding properties of haemoglobin.

Haem biosynthesis

Haem synthesis occurs in the mitochondria by a process outlined in Fig. 4.7.

Haem breakdown

Degradation occurs in the macrophages of the spleen, bone marrow and liver (Fig. 4.8). In haemolytic anaemias, red cells have a shortened lifespan because they are destroyed at an accelerated rate. This

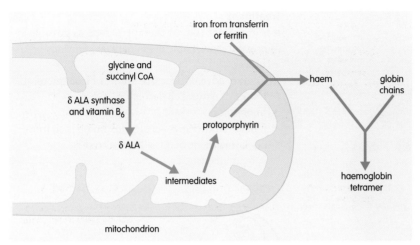

Fig. 4.7 Haem biosynthesis. Glycine and succinyl coenzyme A combine to form δ-aminolaevulinic acid (δ-ALA), a reaction controlled by δ-ALA synthase and the coenzyme vitamin B$_6$. δ-ALA is converted to protoporphyrin, which combines ferrous iron to form haem. The haem molecule combines with a globin chain. Haemoglobin is formed by a tetramer of these haem–globin complexes.

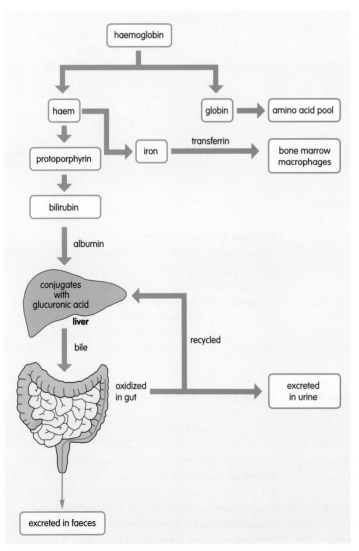

Figure 4.8 Degradation of haemoglobin. Amino acids from the globin chains are recycled to produce new proteins. Iron is transported by transferrin to the bone marrow to produce new erythrocytes. Protoporphyrin is degraded to bilirubin, which is conjugated by the liver and excreted in bile. Bilirubin is excreted in the faeces or converted to urobilinogen, reabsorbed and excreted in the urine.

Fig. 4.9 Clinical features of haemolytic anaemias.

Clinical features of heamolytic anaemias		
Cause	Clinical feature	Mechanism
Increased red-cell destruction	Pallor of mucous membranes	↓ Haemoglobin
	Jaundice	↑ Unconjugated serum bilirubin
	Urine darkens on standing	↑ Urobilinogen
	Pigment gallstones	↑ Bilirubin in bile
	Splenomegaly	↑ Red cell destruction
Increased red-cell production	Folate deficiency	Increased erythropoiesis
	Bone deformities	Erythroid hyperplasia causes expansion of marrow cavities

increased red-cell destruction leads to anaemia, which stimulates increased EPO production, leading to compensatory erythropoiesis. The clinical features of haemolytic anaemias result from the increased red cell-destruction and the compensatory increase in red cell-production (Fig. 4.9).

Haemoglobin

Structure of haemoglobin

Haemoglobin is composed of four globin chains held together by non-covalent interactions (Fig. 4.10). Each chain is associated with a prosthetic haem group, the oxygen-binding site of the molecule. Each globin chain has a hydrophobic crevice, or haem pocket, which contains the haem molecule. Proximal histidine molecules bind to the iron portion of the haem molecule, and distal histidine molecules help stabilize iron in its ferrous state. The haem pocket allows O_2 binding, while protecting the iron atom from oxidation.

Different types of haemoglobin are present at different stages of development (Fig. 4.11). Adult haemoglobin (HbA) contains two α- and two β-chains, which are arranged as two dimers, written $2(\alpha\beta)$. The globin chains interact with each other in an allosteric fashion. Binding of one O_2 increases the affinity for oxygen at the remaining haem groups.

The other major haem-containing protein in humans is myoglobin, which consists of a single chain associated with a haem group. It is found principally in muscle, where it provides an oxygen reserve. The

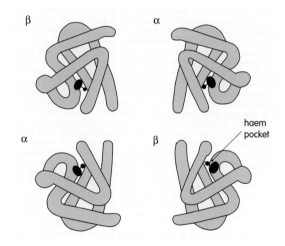

Fig. 4.10 Structure of adult haemoglobin. The α-chain is 141 amino acids long; the β-chain 146 amino acids. A haem pocket can be seen in each globin chain.

four haemoglobin subunits are structurally similar to myoglobin.

Haemoglobin metabolism

The genes encoding the ε-, γ-, δ- and β-chains are found on chromosome 11. The ζ- and two copies of the α-chain genes are found on chromosome 16. The relative positions of these genes are shown in Fig. 4.12. Each globin gene has three exons separated by two introns. The different globin chains are

Haemoglobin during development			
Developmental stage	Haemoglobin type	Chains	Note
Embryonic	Hb Gower I	$\zeta_2\epsilon_2$	
	Hb Gower II	$\alpha_2\epsilon_2$	
	Hb Portland	$\zeta_2\gamma_2$	
Fetal	HbF	$\alpha_2\gamma_2$	Main Hb in later two-thirds of fetal life and in the newborn; higher affinity for O_2 than HbA
Adult	HbA	$\alpha_2\beta_2$	Principal Hb; 68 000 kDa
	HbA_2	$\alpha_2\delta_2$	~2% of adult Hb

Fig. 4.11 Types of haemoglobin present during different stages of development. Hb, haemoglobin; HbA, adult haemoglobin; HbF, fetal haemoglobin.

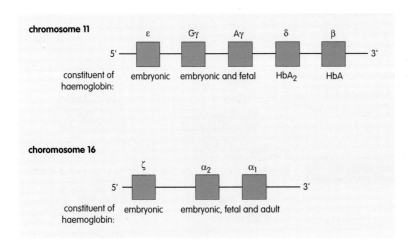

Fig. 4.12 The relative positions of the globin genes. The genes are arranged in the order in which they are expressed during development. The G γ and A γ genes encode γ-chains that differ by just one amino acid. HbA, adult haemoglobin.

synthesized separately and then come together to form a functional Hb molecule.

Physiological properties of haemoglobin

Each haemoglobin molecule (Hb) can bind four molecules of oxygen, one at each haem site. When Hb is oxygenated, relaxed (R-) Hb, the globin chains are able to move against each other, which will allow O_2 release. When O_2 is unloaded, the metabolite 2,3-diphosphoglycerate (2,3-DPG) enters the centre of the deoxyhaemoglobin molecule, reducing its affinity for O_2. Deoxyhaemoglobin, taut (T-) haemoglobin, is characterized by a relatively large number of ionic and hydrogen bonds between the αβ dimers, which restrict the movement of the globin chains.

The oxygen dissociation curve is a plot of partial pressure of oxygen (x axis) against oxygen saturation (y axis) (Fig. 4.13).

The shift of the oxygen dissociation curve to the right in the presence of increased H^+ concentration is called the Bohr effect. This is not the cause of increased ventilatory rate, which is driven by trying to lower CO_2.

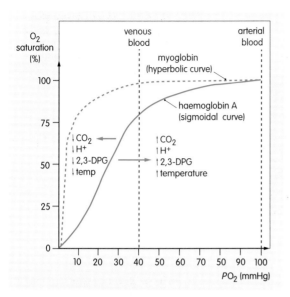

Fig. 4.13 Oxygen dissociation curve for haemoglobin and myoglobin. The haemoglobin curve is sigmoidal in shape because of the cooperative binding of O_2 to haemoglobin. Conversely, unloading of O_2 at one haem group facilitates unloading at the other haem sites. In comparison, the myoglobin curve is hyperbolic in shape, because myoglobin does not release oxygen until the partial pressure of O_2 (pO_2) falls to very low levels. This is because myoglobin does not exhibit cooperative binding. HbA is 100% saturated at a pO_2 of 100 mmHg and 75% saturated at 40 mmHg, the partial pressures of arterial and venous blood respectively. 2,3-DPG, 2,3-diphosphoglycerate.

Changes in CO_2, H^+, 2,3-DPG, and temperature, shift the position of the haemoglobin curve but do not generally alter its shape (Fig. 4.13). H^+ and 2,3-DPG bind to and stabilize deoxyhaemoglobin, favouring the unloading of oxygen. Oxygen binding to myoglobin is not altered by these factors. Haemoglobin variants also have an affect on the oxygen dissociation curve, e.g. sickle-cell haemoglobin shifts the curve to the right. If the curve is shifted to the right, a normal exercise tolerance can be achieved even with a very low haemoglobin count.

High concentrations of 2,3-DPG are present in red cells. During periods of hypoxia, levels of 2,3-DPG are increased, increasing oxygen release in the tissues. Oxygen is transferred from adult to fetal haemoglobin (HbF) because 2,3-DPG binds to HbF less effectively than adult Hb (HbA). In blood stored in acid–citrate–dextrose, red-cell 2,3-DPG levels decline, causing an abnormally high affinity for oxygen and resulting in poor unloading in the tissues.

The cytoskeleton of the red cell

Structure
The erythrocyte plasma membrane is supported by a dense, fibrillar, protein shell—the cytoskeleton. The red-cell cytoskeleton:
- Maintains cell shape and confers strength to the erythrocyte membrane, allowing the cell to withstand the stresses of the circulation
- Permits flexibility, which is important in erythrocyte circulation.

The proteins of the plasma membrane, both integral and peripheral, are important constituents of the cytoskeleton (Fig. 4.14). The band numbers refer to their mobility on electrophoresis.

Integral proteins
Integral proteins penetrate the lipid bilayer and are closely associated with it.

Band 3 protein
Band 3 protein is a glycoprotein homodimer, which transports anions (Cl^-, HCO_3^-). It has binding sites for ankyrin, band 4.1 protein, haemoglobin and glycolytic enzymes. The carbohydrate moiety expresses Ii blood group antigens.

Glycophorins
Glycophorins A, B, C and D are a group of glycoproteins with the same gross structure. Each has three domains: receptor, transmembranous and cytoplasmic.

The cytoplasmic domain of glycophorin A binds cytoskeletal proteins. The receptor domain of glycophorin A has receptors for lectins and influenza virus. Glycophorin A expresses MN blood group antigens, and glycophorin B expresses N, Ss and U blood group antigens.

Peripheral proteins
Peripheral proteins are loosely attached to the lipid bilayer.

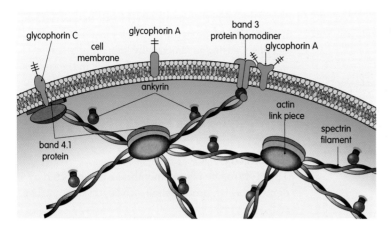

Fig. 4.14 Structure of the red cell cytoskeleton. The hexagonal spectrin lattice is anchored to the membrane by band 3 protein, ankyrin and band 4.1 protein.

Spectrin (bands 1 and 2)

Spectrin is the primary structural component of the cytoskeleton. The α and β subunits of spectrin twist around each other to form heterodimers, which associate to produce tetramers. Tetramers of spectrin are bound together by interactions with band 4.1 protein and actin, to form a hexagonal lattice.

Ankyrin

Ankyrin consists of bands 2.1–2.3 and 2.6. It has binding sites for the β-chain of spectrin and band 3 protein.

Band 4.1 protein

Band 4.1 protein binds spectrin, strengthening the lattice structure. It also binds band 3 protein and glycophorin.

Actin

Actin, also known as band 5, is present in the F actin configuration (short filaments). It binds α- and β-spectrin, supporting the lattice of spectrin tetramers.

The cytoskeleton in disease
Hereditary spherocytosis

This is an autosomal dominant disorder caused by deficiency or dysfunction of one of the skeletal proteins of the erythrocyte membrane. The protein most commonly implicated is spectrin (Fig 4.15). The disordered cytoskeleton network accelerates red-cell destruction, leading to a haemolytic anaemia.

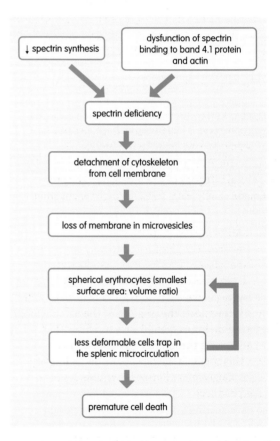

Fig. 4.15 Mechanism of spherocytosis and premature cell death in hereditary spherocytosis due to spectrin deficiency.

Metabolism of red cells

Glucose is the principal energy source for red cells. It is taken up by facilitated diffusion in an insulin-independent fashion. Because red cells have no mitochondria they cannot metabolize glucose aerobically, therefore it is metabolized via:

- The glycolytic pathway (Embden–Meyerhof pathway)
- The hexose monophosphate shunt.

Glycolysis and the Embden–Meyerhof pathway

This is the glycolytic pathway common to all cells of the human body whereby glucose is metabolized to lactate (Fig. 4.16). There is a net yield of two ATP molecules, but no net NADH production.

$$glucose + 2P_i + 2ADP \rightarrow 2\ lactate + 2ATP + 2H_2O$$

Defects of glycolytic enzymes are rare. Approximately 95% are associated with pyruvate kinase and are restricted to red blood cells. Insufficient ATP is produced to maintain the structural integrity of the red cell, leading to premature cell death and a haemolytic anaemia.

The Luebering–Rapoport shunt

This branch of the glycolytic pathway generates 2,3-diphosphoglycerate (2,3-DPG), as illustrated in Fig. 4.17. Trace amounts of 2,3-DPG are found in most cells but high concentrations are found in red cells, where it is important in regulating the affinity of haemoglobin for oxygen. Between 15 and 25% of glucose passing through the glycolytic pathway enters this shunt. In doing so, the reaction catalysed by phosphoglycerate kinase is bypassed, and no net ATP is produced.

The hexose monophosphate shunt

This is also known as the pentose phosphate pathway. Under normal conditions, 5% of the glucose metabolized by the red cell passes through an oxidative pathway of metabolism, the hexose monophosphate (HMP) shunt (Fig. 4.18). There is no net ATP yield, but two NADPH molecules are produced per molecule of glucose-6-phosphate entering the shunt. The majority of the cell's

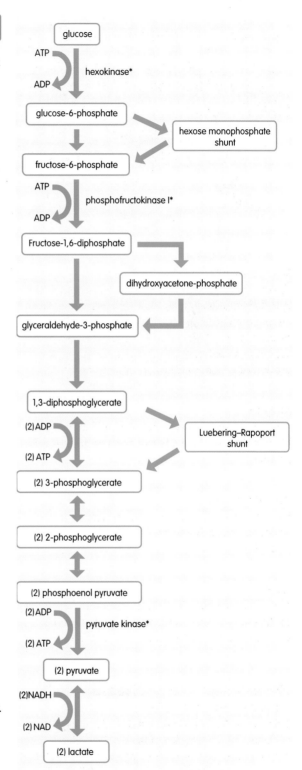

Fig. 4.16 The Embden–Meyerhof pathway. Starred enzymes represent the rate-limiting steps. ADP, adenosine diphosphate; ATP, adenosine triphosphate; NAD/NADH, nicotinamide adenine dinucleotide.

NADPH is produced in this way. NADPH is important in erythrocytes because it reduces oxidized glutathione (GSSG). Reduced glutathione (GSH) is required to maintain sulphydryl groups in their reduced state, which maintains the integrity of haemoglobin and the cytoskeleton.

Glucose-6-phosphate dehydrogenase deficiency is an X-linked disorder characterized by a lack of the enzyme or by a dysfunctional enzyme. Patients are usually asymptomatic, but oxidant stress can induce acute episodes of haemolysis (Fig. 4.19).

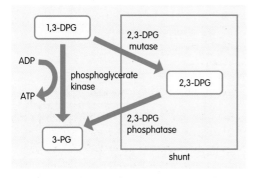

Fig. 4.17 The Luebering–Rapoport shunt. The reaction shown occurs twice per glucose molecule. DPG, diphosphoglycerate; PG, phosphoglycerate.

Prevention of haem oxidation

When haemoglobin is oxidized ($Fe^{2+} \rightarrow Fe^{3+}$) it is known as methaemoglobin (metHb). Excess metHb is caused by:

- Deficiency of reduced nicotinamide adenine dinucleotide (NADH)
- Diaphorase deficiency
- Structurally abnormal Hb (HbM)
- Toxic substances.

The reduced haemoglobin can bind to albumin and has a reduced oxygen-carrying capability. NADH from the Embden–Meyerhof pathway and NADH methaemoglobin reductase are important in ensuring that iron remains in its reduced form.

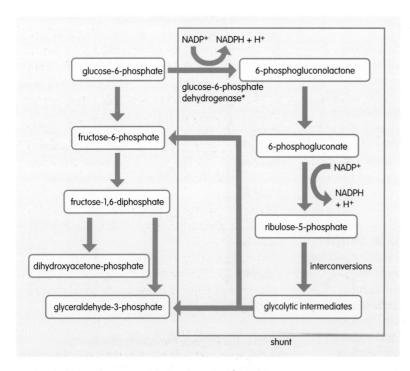

Fig. 4.18 The hexose monophosphate shunt. The first three reactions constitute the irreversible oxidative portion of the pathway and are the sites of NADPH production. The remainder of the pathway is non-oxidative and, in addition to glycolytic intermediates, produces ribulose-5-phosphate, which is used for nucleotide synthesis. The starred enzyme represents the rate-limiting step.

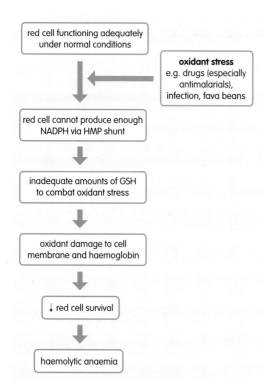

Fig. 4.19 Mechanism of haemolysis in glucose-6-phosphate dehydrogenase deficiency. GSH, reduced glutathione; HMP, hexosemonophosphate; NADPH, nicotinamide adenine dinucleotide phosphate.

Anaemia

Anaemia is a low level of haemoglobin in the blood. Haemoglobin values less than 13 g/dL for men and 12 g/dL for women indicate anaemia, although this does not indicate the need for a blood transfusion.

Anaemia is a common problem worldwide, affecting as much as a third of the world's population. It can be caused by decreased production or increased destruction of erythrocytes, or by blood loss. In developing countries, dietary deficiency and blood loss due to parasitic gut infections are common. In the UK, decreased production is the most common cause.

The physiological response to anaemia attempts to maintain adequate oxygenation of the body. The level of 2,3-DPG rises to ensure that oxygen is unloaded at the tissues. The cardiac output increases and the circulation becomes hyperdynamic. This can be detected by a rapid pulse and heart murmurs. Anaemic patients are often pale. Symptoms vary depending on the cause, but include:

- Fatigue
- Dyspnoea
- Palpitations
- Headache
- Tinnitus
- Anorexia and bowel disturbance.

Anaemias may be classified either morphologically or by cause. Anaemias are micro-, normo- or macrocytic, depending on the mean cell volume (MCV). The mean amount of haemoglobin in each erythrocyte (MCH) is also measured. If the MCH is low, the anaemia is hypochromic.

Anaemia due to impaired red-cell production

Megaloblastic anaemias

In megaloblastic anaemias, impaired DNA synthesis results in the appearance of megaloblasts (abnormal red cell precursors) in the marrow. Megaloblasts are large cells, which contain relatively large abnormal nuclei with finely dispersed chromatin. Anaemia occurs because megaloblasts are removed by bone marrow phagocytes (ineffective erythropoiesis). Megaloblastic anaemia is usually due to deficiency of vitamin B_{12} and/or folate. Both act as coenzymes in the pathway of DNA synthesis. Haematological findings include:

- Macrocytic anaemia (leucopenia and thrombocytopenia in severe megaloblastic anaemia)
- Hypersegmentation of neutrophil nuclei
- Megaloblasts seen on bone marrow smear
- Low serum vitamin B_{12} levels or reduced red cell folate content.

Vitamin B_{12} deficiency

Vitamin B_{12} consists of cobalamin bound to a methyl or adenosyl group. It is found only in foods of animal origin and is not affected by cooking. Absorption occurs in the terminal ileum after combining with intrinsic factor (IF) secreted from gastric parietal cells. Transport within the body is with the plasma-binding protein transcobalamin II.

Vitamin B_{12} is stored in the liver. Body stores are large (~2–3mg), and the daily rate of loss in urine and faeces is small relative to daily requirements (1–2μg); therefore it takes more than 2 years after the onset of the cause of vitamin B_{12} deficiency for anaemia to develop.

Causes of B_{12} deficiency include:
- Dietary, e.g. due to veganism (rare)
- Intrinsic factor deficiency, e.g. congenital, postgastrectomy or due to pernicious anaemia
- Intestinal malabsorption, e.g. due to diseases of the terminal ileum, such as Crohn's disease
- Blind loop or diverticulae in the small bowel that breed bacteria that utilize vitamin B_{12}.

Pernicious anaemia

Pernicious anaemia is an autoimmune chronic atrophic gastritis and is the most common cause of vitamin B_{12} deficiency in adults. Autoantibodies directed against both the gastric parietal cells and IF are detectable in the serum and gastric juice of most patients. Damage to the parietal cells results in failure of IF secretion and vitamin B_{12} absorption. Achlorhydria is an accompanying feature (parietal cells are also responsible for secreting H^+). Pernicious anaemia is associated with autoimmune thyroid disease and patients are at increased risk of gastric carcinoma.

Clinical features of vitamin B_{12} deficiency include:
- A lemon-yellow colour to the skin (if severe), due to a combination of pallor and jaundice
- Glossitis
- Gastrointestinal disturbances
- Weight loss
- Neurological abnormalities (peripheral neuropathy, subacute degeneration of the cord involving the posterior and lateral columns)
- Psychiatric disturbances.

The Schilling test is used to diagnose the cause of vitamin B_{12} deficiency, the steps of which are as follows:
1. Oral, radioactively labelled vitamin B_{12} and intramuscular, non-radioactive vitamin B_{12} are

administered simultaneously. The intramuscular B_{12} saturates the B_{12}-binding proteins in the plasma, promoting urinary excretion of any absorbed radioactive B_{12}
2. The urine is collected for 24 hours after B_{12} administration. If less than 10% of the orally administered B_{12} is excreted, absorption of B_{12} is considered impaired
3. The test is repeated, but this time both oral IF and oral B_{12} are given. If impaired absorption is due to lack of IF (as in pernicious anaemia), B_{12} absorption will be increased. B_{12} absorption will not be increased if the cause of deficiency is malabsorption.

Treatment of vitamin B_{12} deficiency is by correction of the underlying cause, if possible, and intramuscular injections of vitamin B_{12} approximately every 3 months.

Folate deficiency

Folates are derived from folic (pteroyl glutamic) acid. They are found in foods, mainly green vegetables and liver, and are destroyed by cooking. Absorption takes place in the duodenum and jejunum. Folate is stored in the liver. Unlike vitamin B_{12}, folate stores are small (10–15mg) and daily losses are larger relative to daily requirement (100–200μg), therefore a megaloblastic anaemia develops a few months after the onset of folate deficiency.

Causes of folate deficiency are:
- Decreased intake, e.g. due to poor diet
- Decreased absorption, e.g. due to coeliac disease
- Increased requirement due to rapid cell multiplication, e.g. caused by pregnancy, prematurity, malignancy or haemolytic anaemia
- Increased loss, e.g. due to dialysis
- Drugs, e.g. methotrexate (by inhibition of dihydrofolate reductase), anticonvulsants and the oral contraceptive pill.

 Alcohol causes folate deficiency because of malabsorption, malnutrition and increased utilization.

Clinical features of folate deficiency are similar to those of vitamin B_{12} deficiency, without the neurological and psychiatric abnormalities. Treatment of folate deficiency is by correction of any underlying cause and oral supplements of folic acid. If there is a possibility of vitamin B_{12} deficiency, supplements should be given at the same time as folic acid to prevent neurological complications.

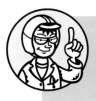 Red cell folate is low in both B_{12} and folate deficiency. A serum folate should be used to differentiate between the two.

Iron-deficiency anaemia

Iron deficiency is the most common cause of anaemia worldwide. It occurs most frequently in women of reproductive age. Anaemia occurs after iron stores have been depleted. Causes of iron-deficiency anaemia include:

- Decreased iron intake, e.g. due to poor diet
- Increased iron requirement, e.g. during growth, pregnancy and lactation
- Chronic blood loss, e.g. due to peptic ulcer
- Decreased iron absorption, e.g. after gastrectomy.

The signs and symptoms of iron-deficiency anaemia (Fig. 4.20) are often only apparent when the haemoglobin level drops below 8g/dL. The haematological findings are:

- A microcytic, hypochromic anaemia
- Reduced serum iron and ferritin (to distinguish from thalassaemia syndromes)
- Increased serum transferrin and total iron-binding capacity (TIBC), (to distinguish from anaemia of chronic disease)
- Reduced plasma transferrin saturation
- Absence of iron stores demonstrated on bone-marrow smear.

Treatment is by oral administration of iron in the form of ferrous sulphate tablets. This must be continued for 4–6 months to replenish iron stores. Any underlying cause should be treated. Parenteral iron is used if the patient has malabsorption or cannot tolerate oral preparations.

Other causes of microcytic anaemia that should be considered are:
- Sideroblastic anaemia (hereditary and acquired). Some respond to vitamin B_6, particularly the former. Vitamin B_6 is a cofactor for haem synthesis, and deficiency prevents iron incorporation. Ringed sideroblasts, red-cell precursors containing iron granules surrounding the nucleus, are seen in the bone marrow (see also p. 78).
- Lead poisoning, which also causes abdominal pain and neuropathy

Fig. 4.20 Signs and symptoms of iron-deficiency anaemia. An atrophic gastritis can also be seen with iron deficiency. In Plummer–Vinson or Paterson–Kelly syndrome, dysphagia and pharyngeal or oesophageal webs accompany the iron deficiency anaemia.

Signs and symptoms of iron-deficiency anaemia	
Features common to other anaemias	**Features specific to iron deficiency**
- Fatigue - Dizziness - Headache - Shortness of breath - Palpitations - Angina - Intermittent claudication - Pallor - Tachycardia - Flow murmur - Congestive cardiac failure	- Glossitis (smooth, sore, red tongue) - Koilonychia (spoon-shaped nails) - Angular stomatitis (sores and cracks at corners of mouth) - Alopecia - Pica (unusual dietary cravings, e.g. for clay and ice)

Anaemia due to increased red-cell destruction (haemolytic anaemias)

Haemolytic anaemias occur when red cell lifespan is reduced. Erythropoiesis can normally be increased seven fold, therefore haemolysis may be compensated and not cause anaemia. Reduced red cell lifespan can be caused by erythrocyte defects or extracorpuscular defects, as shown in Fig. 4.21. It can occur within the circulation or be extravascular:

- **Extravascular haemolysis:** is the route by which red cells are normally broken down and occurs in the macrophages of the spleen, bone marrow and liver
- **Intravascular haemolysis:** is the destruction of red cells within the circulation. It is characterized by all of the features of extravascular haemolysis (see Fig. 4.9, p. 81), as well as by the following:
  - haemoglobinaemia: Hb is released into the bloodstream
  - absence of plasma haptoglobins: Hb binds haptoglobin to form a complex that is removed by macrophages in the reticuloendothelial system
  - haemoglobinuria: the Hb concentration exceeds the tubular reabsorptive capacity and Hb is therefore excreted in the urine

- haemosiderinuria: proximal tubule cells containing intracellular deposits of haemosiderin derived from the Hb reabsorbed in the kidneys are shed in the urine
- methaemalbuminaemia: some of the Hb is oxidized and binds to albumin
- reticulocytosis: erythrocyte precursors enter the blood (also found in extravascular haemolysis).

Hereditary red-cell defects

The defect is usually intrinsic to the red cell, and morphological abnormalities can often be detected on inspection of a peripheral blood smear.

Cytoskeleton defects
Hereditary spherocytosis

Hereditary spherocytosis is a common (prevalence of 1 in 5000 in northern Europe) autosomal dominant disorder of variable penetrance. A defective cytoskeletal protein, most commonly spectrin, causes loss of the membrane. This results in progressive spherocytosis and reduced deformability of red cells, leading to extravascular haemolysis (see Fig. 4.15, p. 84). Haematological findings include:

- Spherocytes on the peripheral blood smear
- Increased osmotic fragility: when suspended in saline solutions of varying concentrations,

Classification of haemolytic anaemias			
Erythrocyte defects		**Extra-corpuscular defects**	
Membrane	Hereditary spherocytosis Hereditary elliptocytosis Paroxysmal nocturnal haemoglobinuria	Immune	Incompatible transfusions Autoimmune haemolytic anaemia Drug associated
Enzyme	G6PD deficiency PK deficiency	Infection	Malaria Septicaemia
Haemoglobin	Sickle-cell syndromes Thalassaemia	Drugs/ chemicals	Dapsone, sulfasalazine
		Mechanical	Microangiopathic haemolysis Prosthetic heart valves DIC, HUS, TTP Following long marches
		Hypersplenism	Myelofibrosis

Fig. 4.21 Classification of haemolytic anaemias. DIC, disseminated intravascular coagulation; G6PD, glucose-6-diphosphate; HUS, haemolytic uraemic syndrome; PK, pyruvate kinase; TTP, thrombotic thrombocytopenic purpura.

spherocytes lyse in less hypotonic solutions than do normal red cells

- Increased autohaemolysis: when spherocytes are incubated in their own plasma, they lyse more readily than normal cells.

The person can be asymptomatic or present at birth with haemolytic disease of the newborn. The usual course is a low-grade anaemia with intermittent 'crises'. Splenectomy can be used to prevent crises and will result in a rise in the Hb level. Pneumococcal, meningococcal and Hib vaccines should be administered before the operation and prophylactic penicillin is recommended postoperatively.

Hereditary elliptocytosis
This autosomal dominant disorder is also due to abnormalities of the cytoskeletal proteins and is most commonly caused by failure of spectrin dimers to form tetramers. It is clinically similar to, but milder than, hereditary spherocytosis. A high proportion of elliptical red cells are seen on the peripheral blood film.

Enzyme defects
Pyruvate kinase deficiency
This is an autosomal recessive condition affecting the glycolytic pathway, which results in a lack of ATP production. Erythrocytes become rigid and are destroyed. The blood film shows a poikilocytosis and distorted 'prickle' cells (seen post-splenectomy). Splenectomy might improve, but not cure, the anaemia.

Glucose-6-phosphate dehydrogenase deficiency
Glucose-6-phosphate dehydrogenase (G6PD) deficiency is an X-linked disorder affecting the hexose monophosphate shunt. There are over 400 variants of G6PD, two of which account for the vast majority of cases: the African (A) and Mediterranean types. Of these two, the Mediterranean type is clinically more severe, because of a much greater reduction in enzyme function. Patients are generally asymptomatic until haemolysis is precipitated by oxidizing factors such as:

- Infection
- Acidosis, e.g. diabetic ketoacidosis
- Drugs, e.g. primaquine, sulphonamides
- Fava beans ('favism'—only in the Mediterranean type).

Haemolysis is primarily intravascular. During a haemolytic crisis, Heinz bodies (precipitates of oxidized, denatured Hb) are generated. Cells that have had Heinz bodies removed upon passing through the spleen, termed 'bite' or 'blister' cells, are seen on the peripheral blood film. Heinz bodies will be seen in patients following splenectomy.

In an asymptomatic patient, the peripheral blood film might be normal. However, G6PD levels are decreased in affected males and carrier females. Assay can be unreliable during or immediately after a haemolytic crisis because reticulocytes (increased in number during a crisis) have higher enzyme levels than mature red cells. In an acute crisis, the precipitating factor should be eliminated and the circulation supported, however, there is no specific treatment.

Other enzyme defects
Several other defects have been identified in enzymes involved in erythrocyte metabolism. They are rare and include hexokinase and glutathione synthetase.

Haemoglobin defects
Thalassaemias

In thalassaemias, there is a defect in the production of the α- or β-globin chains.

β-Thalassaemia occurs most commonly in Mediterranean countries, South-East Asia and Africa. There is a partial or complete failure of β-globin chain production due to:

- Incorrect excision of introns from mRNA (most common)
- Mutations of the regulatory sequences
- Mutations affecting capping
- Mutations affecting polyadenylation of mRNA
- β-Chain gene mutations.

The abnormal β-chain genes are denoted $β^+$ and $β^0$, for partial or complete deficiency respectively. Severity of disease depends on which abnormal genes have been inherited and whether the individual is heterozygous or homozygous.

α-Thalassaemia is most common in South-East Asia and West Africa. There is a deletion of one, two, three or all four α-globin chain genes. The number of deleted genes relates to the severity of disease.

An excess of α-chains (in β-thalassaemia) or β-chains (in α-thalassaemia), results in abnormal aggregation within red-cell precursors, predisposing them to phagocytosis by bone marrow macrophages. Any abnormal red cells that reach the circulation have a shortened lifespan. A number of clinical syndromes are recognized, based on the severity of the anaemia (Fig. 4.22).

β-Thalassaemia major

In β-thalassaemia major, homozygosity for defective genes causes β-chain production to be severely reduced. Investigation reveals:

- Microcytic hypochromic anaemia (Hb 2–3g/dL) and reticulocytosis (at 6–9 months if not transfused)
- Basophilic stippling, target cells and normoblasts on peripheral blood film
- Absence of HbA on electrophoresis
- High serum iron due to increased enteric absorption and regular blood transfusions

- A 'hair-on-end' appearance on skull X-ray (Fig. 4.23). Bony changes are caused by expansion of haemopoietic bone marrow from its normal sites.

Treatment is by regular blood transfusions (about one a month), splenectomy and/or bone marrow transplantation. Chelation therapy is given to prevent iron overload.

β-Thalassaemia minor

This is often known as β-thalassaemia trait because it is heterozygous. Patients are often asymptomatic. Recognition of this syndrome is important as it has implications for genetic counselling and can also mimic iron-deficiency anaemia, for which inappropriate iron therapy might be given.

Sickle-cell syndromes

The sickle Hb (HbS) gene is prevalent in tropical Africa and parts of the Mediterranean, Middle East and India. Up to 40% of the population can be affected in some areas. Sickle-cell trait is thought to afford some protection against *Plasmodium falciparum* malaria, and therefore HbS genes are

Thalassaemia syndromes		
Clinical syndrome	**Type**	**Presentation**
β-thalassaemia major (Mediterranean or Cooley's anaemia)	Homozygous ($\beta^0\beta^0$, $\beta^+\beta^+$, or $\beta^+\beta^0$)	Onset at 6–9 months; severe anaemia, jaundice, failure to thrive, hepatosplenomegaly, bony abnormalities, gallstones, leg ulcers, intercurrent infections
β-thalassaemia intermedia	A variety of genotypes	Presents at 1–2 years of age with a moderate anaemia
β-thalassaemia minor	Heterozygous ($\beta^0\beta$ or $\beta^+\beta$)	Usually asymptomatic; mild microcytic hypochromic anaemia (Hb 10–11g/dL) Raised HbA_2 (4–8% of total Hb)
Silent carrier	3 α genes present	Usually asymptomatic with no detected abnormalities
α-thalassaemia trait	2 α genes present	Normal or slightly low haemoglobin level with microcytic red cells, usually asymptomatic
HbH disease	1 α gene present	Anaemia (7–11g/dL); HbH is formed (β_4) Clinical features of chronic haemolysis
Hydrops fetalis	No α genes present	Fetus usually dies in utero Tetramers of γ-chains form a haemoglobin variant, Hb Barts hydrops Prenatal diagnosis with aggressive transfusions in utero can prevent fetal death

Fig. 4.22 Thalassaemia syndromes. Hb, haemoglobin; HbA, adult haemoglobin; HbF, fetal haemoglobin.

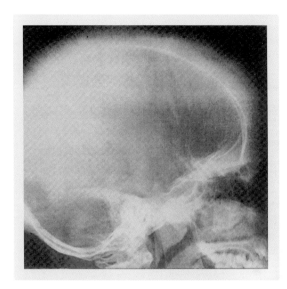

Fig. 4.23 Skull radiograph of a child with β-thalassaemia major. The 'hair-on-end' appearance is pathognomonic. It is caused by extramedullary haemopoiesis.

positively selected in areas where malaria is endemic.

In HbS, a single base-pair substitution in codon 6 of the β-chain replaces glutamic acid with valine. Deoxygenated HbS is 50 times less soluble than deoxygenated HbA and it aggregates and polymerizes to form long intracellular fibres called tactoids. This causes elongation of the red cell into a rigid sickle shape. Reoxygenation can initially reverse the sickling process but, after repeated episodes, the red cells become irreversibly sickled.

HbS polymerizes best with other HbS molecules. The presence of other types of Hb (e.g. HbF or HbA) reduces sickling. Therefore sickle-cell anaemia is not apparent until approximately 6 months of age, when HbF levels fall. Individuals with sickle-cell trait and sickle-cell haemoglobin C disease are asymptomatic or have clinically milder forms of the disease. There are four important syndromes associated with HbS:

1. Sickle-cell anaemia
2. Sickle-cell trait
3. Sickle-cell haemoglobin C disease
4. Sickle-cell β-thalassaemia.

Sickle-cell anaemia (homozygous for HbS, denoted $\beta^s\beta^s$) is the most serious of these. Features of sickle-cell anaemia are listed in Fig. 4.24. Management strategies include:

- Pneumococcal, meningococcal and Hib vaccines
- Penicillin prophylaxis
- Folic acid supplements
- Avoidance of factors precipitating infarctive crises
- Prompt treatment of infection
- Management of infarctive crises with fluids, analgesia (including opiates), warmth and antibiotics if necessary
- Blood transfusions and exchange transfusions when necessary
- Prevention of iron overload.

Sickle-cell trait (heterozygous, HbSA, $\beta^s\beta$) individuals are generally asymptomatic. Sickling occurs at very low partial pressures of oxygen that are rarely reached in vivo. Both HbA and HbS bands are detectable on electrophoresis but sickled cells are not usually seen. Haemoglobin solubility test is positive.

Sickle-cell haemoglobin C disease (HbS/HbC, $\beta^s\beta^c$) arises from carriage of two abnormal β genes. It is clinically similar to, but less severe than, sickle-cell anaemia. Patients are more susceptible to thrombosis and pulmonary embolism and are more likely to develop proliferative retinopathy.

Sickle-cell β-thalassaemia ($\beta^s\beta^0$ or $\beta^s\beta^+$) shares its clinical features with sickle-cell anaemia, but its severity is variable and depends on the amount of normal β-chain synthesis.

Anaemia due to blood loss

Acute blood loss
Causes of acute blood loss include trauma, surgery, peripartum haemorrhage, haematemesis and haemoptysis. Plasma volume is replaced within 1 to 3 days of the acute blood loss but it can take several weeks for the red cell mass, and therefore haemoglobin, to be replenished. Haematological findings in acute blood loss include:

- A normocytic, normochromic anaemia
- A reticulocytosis that peaks 1–2 weeks after the haemorrhage
- An increase in the number of platelets and neutrophils
- Neutrophil precursors in the peripheral blood.

Features of sickle-cell anaemia	
Feature	**Notes**
Chronic haemolytic anaemia	Non-deformable sickled cells are trapped in the splenic microcirculation, leading to premature cell death and the development of pigment gallstones
Infarctive or painful crises	Sickle cells lodge in small and medium sized blood vessels Precipitated by hypoxia, infection, acidosis, dehydration and cold Infected metacarpals and metatarsals cause dactylitis (hand–foot syndrome) in children Chronic tissue and organ damage ensues (bones, lungs, kidneys, liver and brain)
Haemolytic crises	Usually accompany infaractive crises
Aplastic crises	Due to parvovirus infection and to folate deficiency
Spleen	Enlarged in children due to trapped red cells but infarction leads to hyposplenism by ~6 years of age. Before the spleen is destroyed the patient is susceptible to potentially fatal splenic sequestration
Infections	Risk of overwhelming sepsis in early childhood—in asplenic state, more susceptible to infection with encapsulated organisms, e.g. *Streptococcus pneumonia*—prone to *Salmonella* osteomyelitis
Other complications	Priapism, chronic leg ulcers, proliferative retinopathy
Laboratory findings	Hb 6–9 g/dL Reticulocytosis Sickle cells seen on blood film HbS detected on Hb electrophoresis; no HbA Red cells sickle upon mixing with sodium metabisulphite (sickling test) Sickle-cell haemoglobin is insoluble in a high molarity phosphate buffer

Fig. 4.24 Features of sickle-cell anaemia. Hb, haemoglobin; HbA, adult haemoglobin; HbS, sickle haemoglobin.

Red-cell parameters might be normal before compensation for the loss of intravascular volume as both plasma and red cells have been lost in their normal proportions.

Chronic blood loss

The most common causes of chronic blood loss are gastrointestinal lesions and menorrhagia. The consequences are those of iron-deficiency anaemia (see p. 89).

Acquired defects of the red cell
Paroxysmal nocturnal haemoglobinuria

This is a rare, acquired red-cell membrane defect. A mutation in the gene coding for phosphatidylinositol glycan protein A (PIG-A) leads to a lack of glycosyl phosphatidylinositol (GPI). GPI anchors certain proteins to the cell membrane. These proteins usually prevent lysis of blood cells by complement and their absence leads to chronic intravascular haemolysis.

Antibody-mediated red-cell destruction
Autoimmune haemolytic anaemias

In the autoimmune haemolytic anaemias (AIHAs), red-cell autoantibodies cause haemolysis. A positive direct Coombs' test can be demonstrated. There are three types of AIHA:

1. Warm AIHA (occurs at body temperature)
2. Cold AIHA (usually occurs below room temperature)
3. Paroxysmal cold haemoglobinuria.

Warm AIHA can be idiopathic or secondary to autoimmune disease (especially SLE), leukaemias (especially chronic lymphocytic leukaemia), lymphomas and drugs (e.g. methyldopa). The clinical features are as follows:

- Highly variable symptoms that are unrelated to temperature
- Splenomegaly (almost always)

- Evans' syndrome, which is the combination of warm AIHA and idiopathic thrombocytopenic purpura (ITP).

Identified causes should be eliminated. Patients generally respond well to steroids but other immunosuppressive therapies or splenectomy might also be required.

Cold AIHA can be idiopathic or secondary to lymphoma or infection (e.g. mycoplasma pneumonia, Epstein–Barr virus). The clinical features are as follows:

- Symptoms worse in cold weather
- Acrocyanosis (purplish discoloration of the skin) due to vascular sludging arising from red-cell agglutination
- Raynaud's phenomenon.

Treatment involves the elimination of any cause, the patient should be kept warm and immunosuppressive therapy should be considered.

Paroxysmal cold haemoglobinuria is a subset of cold AIHA in which haemolysis occurs at higher temperatures but antibody binding occurs at cold temperatures.

The laboratory features of warm and cold AIHAs are compared in Fig. 4.25.

Alloimmune haemolytic anaemias

Alloimmune haemolytic anaemias are caused by a reaction between antibodies and blood cells from different people. This occurs following:

- transfusion of ABO-incompatible blood
- transfer of maternal antibodies across the placenta in haemolytic disease of the newborn
- allogenic transplantation.

Drug-induced immune haemolytic anaemias

Certain drugs (e.g. penicillin, quinine and methyldopa) can precipitate haemolysis via a variety of immune mechanisms.

Other causes

- Mechanical trauma:
  - microangiopathic haemolytic anaemia occurs when fibrin is deposited in small vessels. This is seen in haemolytic uraemic syndrome, thrombotic thrombocytopaenic purpura, disseminated carcinoma, malignant hypertension and Gram-negative septicaemia. It is characterized by red cell fragments (schistocytes)
  - march haemoglobinuria is caused by damage to red cells in the feet during long periods of walking or running. The blood film does not show fragments
- Chemicals and toxins, e.g. lead poisoning, some snake venoms
- Infection, e.g. malaria
- Hypersplenism.

Features of AIHAs			
Feature	Warm AIHA	Cold AIHA	Paroxysmal cold haemoglobinuria
Antibody class	IgG	IgM	IgG (Donath–Landsteiner)
Antibody specificity	May be Rhesus	May be I or i antigens	Red cell P antigen
Antibody binding temperature	37°C	<32°C	<32°C
Red cell agglutination	✗	✓	✓
Complement fixation	✗	✓	✓
Mechanism of cell destruction	Mainly extravascular	Mainly intravascular	Mainly intravascular
Direct Coombs' test	Positive for IgG and complement	Positive for complement	Positive for IgG and complement

Fig. 4.25 Comparison of laboratory features of autoimmune haemolytic anaemias (AIHAs).

Anaemia of chronic disease

Anaemia of chronic disease results from a multifactorial impairment of erythropoiesis. It is possibly due to a defect in the transfer of iron from the bone marrow macrophages to the red-cell precursors. The anaemia is usually mild to moderate. It is associated with:

- Chronic infections such as tuberculosis and osteomyelitis
- Chronic diseases such as rheumatoid arthritis and SLE
- Malignancies.

Haematological findings include:

- Normocytic, normochromic anaemia or microcytic, hypochromic anaemia
- Reduced serum iron and TIBC (transferrin)
- Normal or high serum ferritin
- Normal or increased bone marrow iron stores.

The last three findings distinguish the microcytic, hypochromic-type from iron-deficiency anaemia. The anaemia does not respond to iron therapy and is correctable only by treatment of the underlying cause. EPO can help to increase erythrocyte production.

Aplastic anaemia

Aplastic anaemia is characterized by pancytopenia and aplasia (hypocellularity) of the bone marrow. There is a reduction in the number of bone-marrow stem cells and those that remain are defective and cannot repopulate the marrow. Causes of aplastic anaemia are listed in Fig. 4.26. Treatment is supportive with removal of any causative factors. Specific treatment is with antilymphocyte globulin,

ciclosporin, haemopoietic growth factors, androgens or stem cell transplantation.

Pure red-cell aplasia

This is a rare condition in which only the red-cell precursors in the bone marrow are defective. Parvovirus B19 causes transient red-cell aplasia.

Other forms of marrow failure

Space-occupying lesions can cause anaemia, e.g. metastatic carcinoma in the bone marrow, which destroys the bone marrow architecture.

Chronic renal failure is almost always associated with anaemia. A decreased renal mass results in reduced production of EPO.

Polycythaemia (erythrocytosis)

Polycythaemia is an increase in haemoglobin concentration above the normal upper limit for the patient's age and sex.

Polycythaemia can be absolute (increased red-cell mass) or relative (reduced plasma volume). The cause of an increased red-cell mass can be primary (in the marrow) or secondary (raised EPO). In conditions causing hypoxia, red-cell mass is increased to raise the oxygen-carrying capacity of blood. This results in an inappropriate rise in EPO. A summary of the causes of polycythaemia is shown in Fig. 4.27.

Causes of aplastic anaemia	
Congenital	**Acquired**
Fanconi type—a rare autosomal recessive condition associated with other congenital anomalies and increased incidence of malignancy	• Idiopathic (50% of cases) • Drugs that cause marrow suppression (e.g. busulphan, chloramphenicol) • Ionizing radiation • Chemicals, e.g. benzene, insecticides • Infection, e.g. viral hepatitis

Fig. 4.26 Causes of aplastic anaemia.

Fig. 4.27 Causes of polycythaemia.

Causes of polycythaemia	
Absolute	**Relative**
Primary • Polycythaemia rubra vera (see text)	Fluid depletion • Dehydration (diarrhoea and vomiting) • Plasma loss, e.g. burns Cigarette smoking Stress (associated with smoking, alcohol, hypertension, obesity, diuretic therapy)
Secondary Appropriately increased erythropoietin: • High altitude • Chronic lung disease • Cyanotic heart diseases • Haemoglobin with abnormally high O_2 affinity Inappropriately increased erythropoietin: • Renal disease (carcinoma, cysts, transplants) • Hepatocellular carcinoma • Cerebellar haemangioblastoma • Massive uterine fibroids	

Primary polycythaemia (polycythaemia rubra vera)

An abnormal clone of stem cells gives rise to increased numbers of red cells, neutrophils and platelets. The red-cell precursors are inappropriately sensitive to insulin-like growth factor +/− interleukin-3 and therefore do not require EPO to avoid apoptosis. Presentation is most commonly due to symptoms of vascular occlusion. Haematological findings include:

• Raised packed cell volume, red-cell mass, haemoglobin and red-cell count
• Raised white-cell count (neutrophils and basophils)
• Raised neutrophil alkaline phosphatase
• Raised platelet count
• Hyperplasia of erythroid, granulocytic and megakaryocytic cells in bone marrow
• Decreased serum EPO
• Increased plasma urate
• Increased total blood volume and blood viscosity.

Treatment is by venesection. Other therapies include cytotoxic drugs (such as hydroxyurea) and irradiation of the bone marrow using [32]P. Some patients develop acute leukaemia or myelofibrosis. The main causes of death are thromboses and acute leukaemia. However, if the red-cell count is kept low, the prognosis is good.

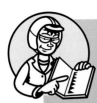

- What changes occur to cells during erythropoiesis?
- How is erythropoietin controlled?
- How is the erythrocyte specialized for its functions?
- What processes allow carbon dioxide to be transported from the tissues to the lungs?
- What are the consequences of excess iron in the body and how can it be treated?
- How does the breakdown of haemoglobin relate to the clinical features of haemolytic anaemias?
- What defects cause the thalassaemias and sickle-cell disease?
- Why is the oxygen dissociation curve sigmoidal, what factors affect its position and why is shifting the curve important in hypoxia?
- How is iron taken up, transported and excreted?
- What is the pathway of glucose metabolism in erythrocytes?
- Why are the Luebering–Rapoport and hexose monophosphate shunts important for red cell functioning?
- Why might chronic renal failure cause anaemia and how is this anaemia treated?
- What conditions result in a normocytic anaemia?
- What red-cell cytoskeletal defects are most common and why do they lead to haemolysis?
- What are the differences between warm and cold autoimmune haemolytic anaemia?
- What is aplastic anaemia and what are the causes?
- Why might a person have polycythaemia?
- How does sickle-cell anaemia present?
- What features occur in the different α-thalassaemias?
- What factors can precipitate a haemolytic crisis in a patient with glucose-6-phosphate dehydrogenase deficiency?

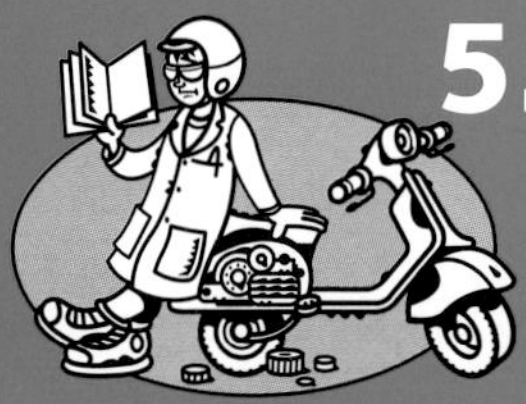

5. White Blood Cells

Structure and function of the white blood cells

See Chapter 1 for a discussion of the immunological functions of white blood cells.

Lymphocytes
Appearance and structure
Lymphocytes Fig. 5.1 are the smallest white cells, 6–15 μm in diameter. In blood they are round but they can change shape outside the circulation. They have round, densely staining, acentric nuclei. The sparse cytoplasm contains a few lysosome-like granules. Once activated, the amount of cytoplasm increases. B cells and natural killer (NK) cells tend to be larger than T cells. The cells are differentiated by the presence of differing surface markers.

Location
Lymphocytes circulate between tissue, lymphatics and the blood. The lifespan of lymphocytes varies depending on their interaction with antigens. Memory cells can survive for decades.

Function
Lymphocytes have no functions in the blood, but are central to the adaptive immune response. They produce antibodies and kill foreign or virally altered cells.

Neutrophils
Appearance and structure
Neutrophils (Fig. 5.2), also known as polymorphonuclear leucocytes, measure 9–15 μm in diameter. They have distinctive nuclei containing 2–5 lobes connected by thin chromatin threads. In females, the nucleus has a 'drumstick' appendage that contains the inactivated X chromosome. Neutrophils have few mitochondria and large stores of glycogen. The cytoplasm contains an abundance of three types of granule:

1. Small, specific granules (0.1 μm in diameter) containing antimicrobial enzymes and other agents
2. Azurophilic granules (0.5 μm in diameter) similar to lysosomes
3. Tertiary granules containing gelatinase, cathepsins and glycoproteins.

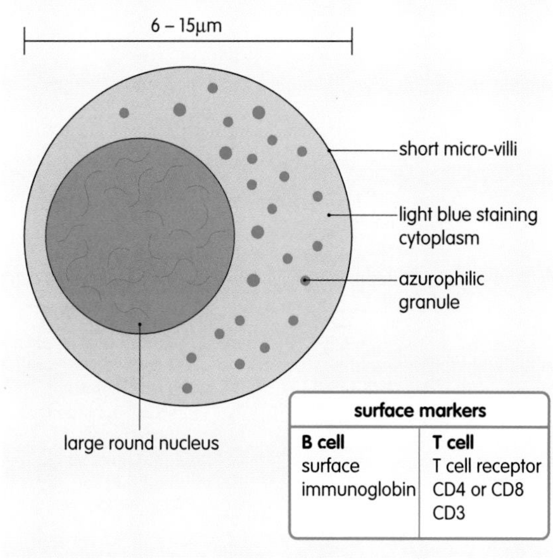

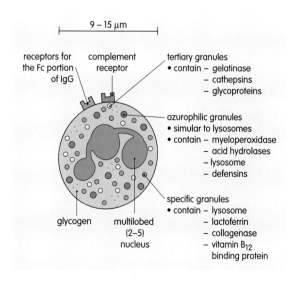

Fig. 5.1 Lymphocyte structure.

Fig. 5.2 Neutrophil structure.

Location

Neutrophils circulate in blood for up to 10 hours. In response to chemotactic agents they migrate into tissues, where they survive for 1–3 days.

Function

Neutrophils are the first cells to reach sites of inflammation and, once defunct, they are the major constituent of pus. They destroy microorganisms by phagocytosis and release of hydrolytic enzymes.

Monocytes
Appearance and structure

Monocytes (Fig. 5.3) tend to be the largest circulating blood cell, up to 25 μm diameter. They have a large, kidney-shaped nucleus. Nucleoli are often present, giving the nucleus a 'moth-eaten' appearance. The cytoplasm contains many lysosomes and vacuole-like spaces producing a 'ground-glass' appearance. Microtubules, microfilaments, pinocytotic vesicles and filo- or pseudopodia are present around the edge of the cell.

Location

Monocytes spend only a few days in the blood before migrating into the tissues, where they differentiate to become macrophages. Macrophages survive for several months to years in connective tissue.

Function

Monocytes form the reticuloendothelial system, which is primarily involved in phagocytosis. They destroy dead or defunct cells and ingest foreign material. Antigens are processed and can be presented to lymphocytes to initiate an adaptive immune response. Macrophages also have a proinflammatory function, releasing a variety of cytokines.

Eosinophils
Appearance and structure

Eosinophils (Fig. 5.4) are similar to neutrophils but larger: 12–17 μm diameter. Their nucleus is sausage-shaped and usually bilobed. They have a small, central Golgi apparatus and limited rough endoplasmic reticulum and mitochondria. Eosinophils contain large, ovoid, specific granules and azurophilic granules. The specific granules (1–1.5 μm long) have a crystalloid centre containing major basic protein, eosinophilic cationic protein and eosinophil-derived neurotoxin. The outside of the granule contains several enzymes, including histaminase, peroxidase and cathepsin.

Location

They are primarily found in the tissues, spending less than 1 hour in blood.

Function

Their primary function is to combat parasitic infection. Eosinophils also phagocytose antigen–antibody complexes.

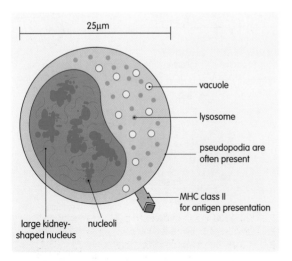

Fig. 5.3 Monocyte structure. MHC, major histocompatibility complex.

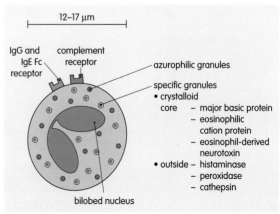

Fig. 5.4 Eosinophil structure.

Basophils

Appearance and structure

Basophils (Fig. 5.5) are 14–16μm diameter with a bilobed 'S-shaped' nucleus. They are named after their highly basophilic cytoplasmic specific granules, but also contain azurophilic granules. Specific granules (0.5μm in diameter) are large, membrane-bound round or oval structures. They push into the plasma membrane causing a 'roughened perimeter'. The granules contain heparin, histamine, chemotactic factors and peroxidase.

Location

The lifespan is unknown, however they survive for 1–2 years in mice.

Function

It is not clear whether basophils are the precursors to mast cells, with which they share many similarities. Basophils are thought to mediate inflammatory responses.

Differentiation of white cells

Granulocytes and monocytes are formed in the bone marrow from a common precursor cell (CFU-GM). Their differentiation pathways are shown in Fig. 5.6.

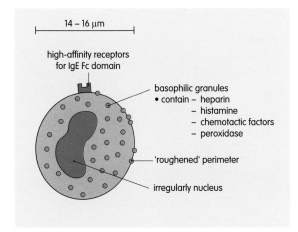

Fig. 5.5 Basophil structure.

Reactive proliferation of white cells

Leucocytosis

Leucocytosis is an increase in the total white cell count ($>11 \times 10^9$/L). Figure 5.7 outlines the numerical criteria for normal differential white-cell counts. One leucocyte type, most commonly

Increased granulocyte counts are known as neutrophilia, eosinophilia or basophilia, whereas raised non-granulocyte levels are referred to as lymphocytosis or monocytosis.

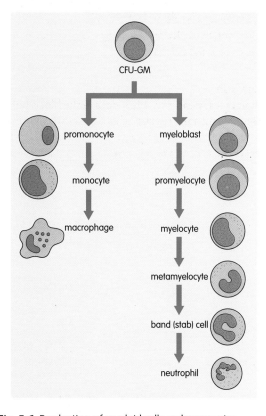

Fig. 5.6 Production of myeloid cells and monocytes. Eosinophils and basophils are formed by a process similar to the one shown for neutrophils. Neutrophils usually develop within bone marrow, but with increased demand, e.g. severe infection, band cells may be seen in blood. CFU-GM, granulocyte, monocyte colony-forming unit.

Differential white-cell counts	
Cell type	Normal levels
Leucocytes	$4-11 \times 10^9/L$
Neutrophils	$2-7.5 \times 10^9/L$
Eosinophils	$0.04-0.44 \times 10^9/L$
Basophils	$0-0.1 \times 10^9/L$
Lymphocytes	$1.3-3.5 \times 10^9/L$
Monocytes	$0.2-0.8 \times 10^9/L$

Fig. 5.7 Normal values for differential white-cell counts. Normal black and Middle Eastern people may have lower counts. Children younger than 12 years of age and pregnant women normally exhibit higher levels of white cells.

neutrophils, tends to predominate, with small increases in other types. Diseases associated with increases in white-cell count are listed in Fig. 5.8.

Lymphadenopathy

The lymph nodes can become enlarged during any infective or inflammatory disease, but can be an important indicator of haematological disease. Acute presentation of rapidly expanding painful nodes is likely to be infectious. Slow growth of painless nodes is often haematological in origin. If lymphadenopathy is localized, the cause is more likely to be localized. Common causes of lymphadenopathy are shown in Fig. 5.9.

Fig. 5.8 Diseases associated with increased white-cell counts. TB, tuberculosis.

Diseases associated with increases in white-cell count		
Cell type	Associated diseases	Examples
Leucocytes	Pathological stress, leukaemia	
Neutrophils	Bacterial infections	Pyogenic bacteria
	Acute inflammation or tissue necrosis	Infarction, surgery, burns, myositis, vasculitis
	Neoplasms	Carcinoma, lymphoma, melanoma
	Myeloproliferative disorders	Chronic myeloid leukaemia, myelofibrosis
	Metabolic disorders	Eclampsia, gout, diabetic ketoacidosis
Eosinophils	Parasitic infestation	Malaria, hookworm, filariasis, schistosomiasis
	Allergic reaction	Asthma, hay fever
	Skin disease	Pemphigus, eczema, psoriasis, dermatitis herpetiformis, urticaria
	Neoplasms	Hodgkin's disease, metabolic carcinoma, chronic myeloid leukaemia
	Infections	Convalescent phase of any infection
Basophils	Myeloproliferative disorders	Chronic myeloid leukaemia, polycythaemia rubra vera
Lymphocytes	Acute infections	Infectious mononucleosis, pertussis, rubella, viral infection
	Chronic infections	TB, syphilis
	Neoplasms	Chronic lymphocytic leukaemia, lymphoma
Monocytes	Chronic infections and inflammatory diseases	TB, bacterial endocarditis, protozoa
	Neoplasms	Lymphomas, myelodysplastic syndromes

Fig. 5.9 Causes of lymphadenopathy. HIV, human immunodeficiency virus.

Causes of lymphadenopathy	
Cause	**Example**
Infective	*Streptococcus* spp.
	Mycobacterium tuberculosis
	Epstein–Barr virus
	HIV
	Toxoplasmosis
	Brucellosis
	Histoplasmosis
	Coccidioidomycosis
Neoplasia	Leukaemias
	Lymphomas
	Secondary, e.g. lung, breast
Connective tissue disease	Rheumatoid arthritis
	Systemic lupus erythematosus
Drugs	Phenytoin
	Para-aminosalicylic acid
Others	Sarcoidosis
	Amyloidosis

Fig. 5.10 Possible differentiation pathways of multipotent myeloid stem cells and associated myeloproliferative disorders.

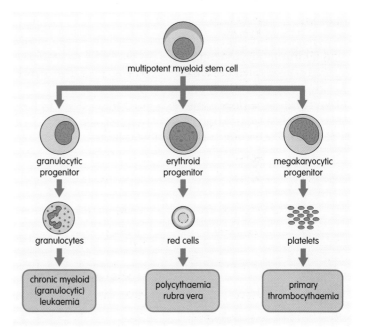

Neoplastic proliferation of white cells

Myeloproliferative disorders

These disorders arise as a result of the neoplastic clonal proliferation of multipotent myeloid stem cells, which are capable of following one or more differentiation pathways (Fig. 5.10).
Myeloproliferative disorders encompass:

- Chronic myeloid leukaemia (see p. 106)
- Primary polycythaemia (polycythaemia rubra vera) (see p. 97)
- Myelofibrosis
- Primary thrombocythaemia.

Myelofibrosis

Chronic idiopathic myelofibrosis is also known as agnogenic myeloid metaplasia. It can be preceded by other myeloproliferative conditions. Bone marrow is replaced by fibrous tissue, produced by fibroblasts, in conjunction with the proliferation of dysplastic megakaryocytes. Massive splenomegaly occurs due to extramedullary haemopoiesis. The disease affects individuals from middle-age onwards. Features at presentation include anaemia, leucocytosis and thrombocytosis. Blood films reveal:

- Granulocyte precursor cells
- Nucleated red blood cell precursors
- Tear-drop poikilocytosis (tear-drop-shaped erythrocytes).

Supportive care including transfusions of red cells can be useful, and splenectomy or splenic irradiation are sometimes beneficial. Chemotherapy with hydroxyurea can slow or reverse fibrosis. Median survival is 3 years. Approximately 10% of cases transform into acute myeloblastic leukaemia (AML).

Primary thrombocythaemia

A raised platelet count (>600 × 10^9/L) is the dominant feature. It usually presents after the age of 50 but the incidence is increasing in younger women. About half of affected individuals are asymptomatic at diagnosis. The disorder is characterized clinically by thrombosis or bleeding. Haemorrhage is more common with higher platelet counts, e.g. >1000 × 10^9/L, and in those with acquired von Willebrand's disease (see p. 126). There are raised levels of abnormal megakaryocytes in the bone marrow. Splenic atrophy, as a result of microinfarcts, occurs in 50% of cases. Treatment involves the reduction of platelet levels by hydroxyurea or anegrelide. Aspirin is commonly used to reduce thrombotic risk.

Neoplasia of myeloid origin
Myelodysplastic syndromes

Myelodysplasias are acquired neoplastic disorders of the bone marrow. A defect in myeloid precursors causes bone marrow failure and abnormalities of red cells, granulocytes, monocytes and platelets. Common features of myelodysplasias include:

- Normal or increased bone marrow cellularity
- Cytopenias
- Occurs most commonly in the elderly and males
- Progression to AML
- Often follows chemo- and/or radiotherapy for another condition
- Slowly progressing disease often with anaemia, easy bruising or bleeding and infections.

The five myelodysplastic syndromes are classified in Fig. 5.11. Survival is best when blasts occupy less than 5% of the marrow.

Classification of myelodysplastic syndromes		
Type	Peripheral blood	Bone marrow
Refractory anaemia (RA)	Blasts <1%	Blasts <5%
Refractory anaemia with ringed sideroblasts (RARS)	Blasts <1%	Blasts <5%, ring sideroblasts >15% of total erythroblasts
RA with excess blasts (RAEB)	Blasts <5%	Blasts 5–20%
RAEB in transformation*	Blasts >5%	Blasts 20–30% or Auer rods present
Chronic myelomonocytic leukaemia (CMML)	Any above + >1.0 × 10^9/L monocytes	Any above + promomonocytes

*Now often considered to be acute myeloid leukaemia.

Fig. 5.11 The French-American-British (FAB) classification of myelodysplastic syndromes.

Leukaemias

Leukaemias are a group of disorders characterized by accumulation of abnormal blood cells in bone marrow. They are clonal disorders, i.e. they result from successive uncontrolled divisions of a single cell. The leukaemic 'blast' cells are non-functional and replace normal bone marrow, encroaching on normal haemopoietic cell development. This leads to:

- Anaemia
- Neutropenia
- Thrombocytopenia.

Many symptoms of leukaemia are due to organ infiltration by leukaemic cells. Organs that are commonly involved include:

- Bones.
- Lymph nodes.
- Liver and spleen (might also be involved by extramedullary haemopoiesis).
- Skin.
- Central nervous system.

Classification of leukaemia is based on:

- Cell lineage (lymphoid or myeloid)
- Developmental stage of leukaemic cells: acute leukaemia involves proliferation of immature cells (blasts) and, untreated, is usually rapidly fatal; chronic leukaemia involves more mature cells, and a more prolonged course is characteristic.

Acute leukaemias are myeloblastic (AML) or lymphoblastic (ALL). The French–American–British (FAB) classification (Fig. 5.12) further subdivides acute leukaemia into different groups based on their morphology and cytochemistry.

Acute myeloblastic leukaemia

Acute myeloblastic leukaemia (AML) is characterized by a rapidly progressive accumulation of primitive myeloblasts in bone marrow and peripheral blood. The incidence increases with age (median 60 years), with an average of 1 in 10000 per year. The 5-year survival rate is about 50%. AML is associated with:

- Radiation exposure
- Toxins: benzene, alkylating agents
- Hereditary abnormalities, e.g. Down syndrome
- Pre-existing haematological disease: chronic myeloid leukaemia (CML), myelodysplastic syndromes.

FAB classification of acute leukaemia	
Myeloblastic	**Lymphoblastic**
M0—undifferentiated myeloblastic leukaemia	L1—homogeneous population of small lymphoblasts
M1—acute myeloblastic leukaemia without maturation	L2—heterogeneous population of large lymphoblasts with one or more nucleoli
M2—acute myeloblastic leukaemia with maturation	L3—homogeneous population of large lymphoid cells with basophilic, vacuolated cytoplasm (now known as Burkitt's leukaemia/lymphoma)
M3—acute promyelocytic leukaemia	
M4—acute myelomonocytic leukaemia	
M5—acute monoblastic leukaemia	
M6—acute erythroleukaemia	
M7—acute megakaryoblastic leukaemia (rare)	

Fig. 5.12 The French–American–British (FAB) classification of acute leukaemias.

Patients are often acutely unwell at presentation and can present with:
- Anaemia, malaise, sweats, weight loss
- Infections (chest, mouth, skin)
- Bleeding
- Skin infiltration (gums M4/5)
- Leucostasis.

Leucostatic symptoms occur when white blood cells form thrombi in the heart, lungs and brain. Symptoms include reduced consciousness, retinal haemorrhages and pulmonary infiltrates.

Chromosome rearrangements have prognostic value with t(15;17), t(8;21) and inversion of 16 having better outcomes than monosomy 7.

AML is treated with combination chemotherapy (as part of national trials by the Medical Research Council) and, in some cases, bone marrow transplantation; 35% of people can be cured by chemotherapy alone, rising to 45% with bone marrow transplant. Survival is best in younger patients. The haematological consequences of AML are treated to improve symptoms and outcome. This includes transfusions of red cells/platelets, leukopheresis to reduce blood viscosity and the prevention/treatment of infection.

Chronic myeloid leukaemia
CML, also known as chronic granulocytic leukaemia, is a progressive accumulation of mature myeloid cells in blood and bone marrow. At presentation the white-cell count can be $300-500 \times 10^9$/L (normal levels are between 4 and 11×10^9/L). It accounts for 20% of all leukaemias. The average incidence is 1 in 100000, peaking between 40 and 60 years of age. It is rare in children and there is a slight male preponderance. Clinically, there are three phases of disease:
1. Chronic
2. Accelerated
3. Blast crisis (AML/ALL).

People normally present in the chronic phase following an incidental finding on a full blood count or with constitutional (malaise, weight loss, sweats) or leucostatic symptoms. Most patients will quickly transform to an accelerated or blast crisis stage.

A disease marker, the Philadelphia chromosome, denoting a (9;22) translocation is found in granulocytic, erythrocytic and megakaryocytic precursor cells. This translocation fuses parts of two genes (BCR-ABL) to create an abnormal tyrosine kinase, which is thought to be involved in disease progression. A tyrosine kinase inhibitor STI 571 (traded as Glivec) is now available, which has improved outcome for these patients. Bone marrow transplantation is potentially curative.

Median survival is $5\frac{1}{2}$ years. Good prognostic factors include:
- Youth
- Small spleen at presentation
- Low white-cell count at presentation.

Neoplasia of lymphoid origin
Acute lymphoblastic leukaemia
ALL accounts for 80% of all childhood leukaemias but is rare in adults. The peak incidence occurs between 2 and 10 years of age. Presentation outside of this range confers a poorer prognosis. ALL is associated with:
- Radiation
- Chemicals
- Down syndrome
- Fanconi's syndrome.

In 80% of cases, the blast cells are of B cell origin. ALL is more responsive to combination chemotherapy than AML and remission rates of 70% are attained. Cure rates are highest in females under 5 years old. The Philadelphia chromosome is seen in 10–20% of cases and is associated with a poor outcome.

Chronic lymphocytic leukaemia
CLL occurs most frequently in people over the age of 60 years (median age 65) and accounts for 20–50% of all leukaemias. It is twice as common in men than women, with a total incidence of 3–4 per 10000. CLL arises from a proliferation of neoplastic lymphoid cells (B cells), which infiltrate the marrow, lymph nodes, spleen and liver. It is a slowly progressing, low-grade disorder. Symptoms seen in other leukaemias are seen in 50% of CLL at diagnosis

and associated autoimmune haemolytic anaemia is common.

On a blood film, leukaemic cells resemble mature lymphocytes, although typical 'smear cells' are also seen. Disease transformation into acute leukaemia does not occur. Median survival is 5–8 years and treatment (chemotherapy or stem cell transplantation) is usually aimed at limiting rather than curing the disease. Many elderly patients will die of an unrelated condition because of the slow nature of the disease.

Hairy cell leukaemia

This condition causes a pancytopenia due to a monoclonal proliferation of a type of B cell with an irregular cytoplasmic outline. The number of 'hairy' cells in the peripheral blood is very variable, however, they are found in bone marrow. The peak incidence is 40–60 years of age, with males four times more likely than females to develop hairy cell leukaemia. Treatment with 2-chlorodeoxyadenosine or deoxycoformycin causes remission in >90% of cases.

Malignant lymphomas

Lymphomas are a group of neoplastic disorders characterized by the proliferation of a primitive cell to produce a clonal expansion of lymphoid cells. They primarily involve the lymph nodes and extranodal lymphoid tissue, e.g. mucosal-associated lymphoid tissue (MALT) and spleen.

Malignant lymphomas are divided into two categories:

1. Non-Hodgkin's lymphoma
2. Hodgkin's disease (Hodgkin's lymphoma).

Although it is easy to think of leukaemias as disease of the bone marrow, and lymphomas as disease of the lymph nodes, remember that leukaemic cells are found in the blood and that lymphoma cells commonly spread to the bone marrow and blood.

Non-Hodgkin's lymphomas

Non-Hodgkin's lymphomas (NHL) are a group of malignant diseases involving lymphoid cells. NHL is classified into low-, intermediate- and high-grade disease in terms of clinical behaviour (Fig. 5.13). Incidence of NHL rises with age and is more common in men than women. There are several aetiological factors associated with NHL including:

- Infections, e.g. Epstein–Barr virus and human T cell lymphotrophic virus 1
- Immunodeficiency, e.g. immunosuppressive therapy, HIV

Fig. 5.13 The Revised American European Lymphoma (REAL) classification of non-Hodgkin's lymphoma.

	REAL classification of non-Hodgkin's lymphoma	
Grade	**B cell**	**T cell**
Low	Small lymphocytic lymphoma Lymphoplasmacytic lymphoma/ Waldenstrom's macroglobulinaemia Marginal zone lymphomas Follicular lymphoma (grades I and II)	Sezary's syndrome/mycosis fungoides Smouldering/chronic adult T cell leukaemia/ lymphoma
Intermediate	Mantle cell lymphoma Follicular lymphoma (grade III)	Peripheral T cell lymphoma Angioimmunoblastic lymphoma Angiocentric lymphoma Intestinal T cell lymphoma
High	Diffuse large B cell lymphoma Primary mediastinal B cell lymphoma Precursor B lymphoblastic Burkitt's lymphoma	Anaplastic lsarge cell lymphoma Precursor T lymphoblastic Adult T cell leukaemia/lymphoma

- Autoimmune disorders
- Irradiation and carcinogens
- Inherited disorders, e.g. ataxia telangiectasia, Fanconi's syndrome.

The incidence of NHL has increased since the 1970s, probably because of increases in the number of immunodeficient people. The features of NHL are outlined in Fig. 5.14.

Low-grade lymphomas

Follicle centre cell lymphomas are the most common type. Low-grade disease has a benign course and responds to treatment. It is difficult to eradicate and relapse is inevitable. Chemotherapy and monoclonal antibody therapy are often used. Survival is 7–10 years and patients tend to die from resistant disease, infection or transformation to a higher-grade lymphoma.

Intermediate-grade lymphomas

Mantle cell lymphomas are increasingly recognized as being intermediate grade. They do not respond well to treatment but progress rapidly (median survival 3 years).

High-grade lymphomas

Large cell lymphomas are the most common. They respond well to treatment (40–50% long-term survival) if localized but otherwise they are aggressive and rapidly progressive. The standard treatment regimen is known as CHOP (cyclophosphamide, adriamycin, vincristine and prednisolone).

Hodgkin's disease

Hodgkin's disease (HD) characteristically affects young males in the third and fourth decades of life. There is a second peak of incidence in the elderly. Diagnosis requires the presence of pathognomonic Reed–Sternberg (RS) cells or derivatives, typically mixed with a variable inflammatory infiltrate. Disease severity is directly proportional to the number of RS cells found in the lesions and indirectly linked to the number of lymphocytes in the lesions. The RS cells are neoplastic derivatives of B cells with a dysfunctional immunoglobulin gene. RS cells are bi- or multinucleated, with prominent eosinophilic nucleoli, giving an 'owl's-eye' appearance. The clinical features of HD are shown in Fig. 5.15.

Hodgkin's disease has been classified into four histological subtypes (Fig. 5.16). Although

---

Features of non-Hodgkin's lymphoma

- Superficial, asymmetric, painless lymphadenopathy
- Fever, night sweats and weight loss
- Oropharyngeal involvement (5–10%)
- Cytopenias due to marrow failure or autoimmunity
- Abdominal disease (spleen, liver, MALT and retroperitoneal/mesenteric nodes)

Fig. 5.14 Features of non-Hodgkin's lymphoma. MALT, mucosal-associated lymphoid tissue.

Clinical features of Hodgkin's disease

Painless, non-tender lymphadenopathy: cervical then axillary nodes are most common, mediastinal in 10%
Splenomegaly (rarely massive)
Respiratory symptoms (mediastinal mass → Superior vena cava obstruction)
Pruritus
Constitutional symptoms
- Weight loss
- Sweats
- High swinging 'Pel-Ebstein' fever
- Alcohol-induced pain

Fig. 5.15 Clinical features of Hodgkin's disease.

Fig. 5.16 Rye classification of Hodgkin's disease (HD). RS, Reed–Sternberg.

Rye classification of Hodgkin's disease (HD)	
Lymphocyte predominant	10% of cases of HD. The infiltrate consists of large numbers of lymphocytes and histiocytes, interspersed with a few RS cells. This subtype has a good prognosis
Nodular sclerosing	50% of cases of HD and, unlike other forms of HD, is more common in women. Broad bands of collagen fibres divide the lymph node into nodules containing a mixture of lymphocytes, eosinophils, plasma cells, macrophages and lacunar cells
Mixed cellularity	30% of cases of HD. It is characterized by an infiltrate of histiocytes, plasma cells and eosinophils. Fewer lymphocytes and more RS cells are present than in the lymphocyte-predominant form of the disease
Lymphocyte depletion	10% of cases of HD. RS cells or their variants are present in large numbers in conjunction with relatively few lymphocytes. Lymphocyte depletion has the poorest prognosis of all forms of HD

Fig. 5.17 Ann Arbor staging of malignant lymphomas.

Ann Arbor staging of malignant lymphomas	
Stage	**Sites of involvement**
I	Disease limited to single region of nodes or one extranodal site
II	Disease at two sites on the same side of the diaphragm
III	Disease at several sites on both sides of the diaphragm (includes spleen)
IV	Spread of disease to extra lymphatic structures, e.g. bone marrow, gut, lung, liver

A: no symptoms
B: weight loss, sweats, fever

histological composition is an important prognostic factor, clinical staging (Ann-Arbor staging) is the most accurate indicator of long-term prognosis in HD (Fig. 5.17). Treatment depends on stage. Stages 1A and 2A receive radiotherapy, which cures 75–95%. Other stages receive combination chemotherapy over 6 months but only 50–65% are cured. Late complications of the disease include:
• Infertility
• Radiation pneumonitis
• Pulmonary fibrosis
• Secondary cancers, including AML.

Multiple myeloma
Multiple myeloma is a malignant proliferation of plasma cells in bone marrow, which produce a monoclonal paraprotein and/or light chain. The monoclonal immunoglobulin is found in serum, whereas the light-chain or Bence-Jones protein is found in urine. These monoclonal proteins form a discrete band on the electrophoretic strip (Fig. 5.18).

The incidence of multiple myeloma is 4–6/100000 a year. It is a disease of late middle age and the elderly. Survival with adequate treatment (combination chemotherapy, thalidomide, localized radiotherapy) is 3–5 years. The aetiology is unknown, apart from an increased incidence related to exposure to ionizing radiation. Tumour necrosis factor and interleukin-6 have been implicated in initiation of disease.

Diagnosis requires:
• Monoclonal paraprotein in serum or urine
• >10–15% of bone marrow to be plasma cells
• Osteolytic bone lesions on skeletal survey.

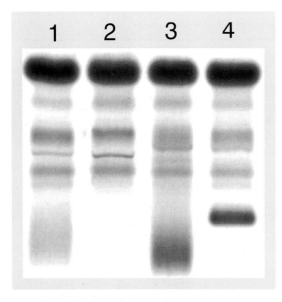

Fig. 5.18 Serum electrophoresis. Lane 1, normal sample; lane 2, patient with antibody deficiency; lane 3, patient with infection and polyclonal raised immunoglobulins; lane 4, patient with myeloma and monoclonal immunoglobulin.

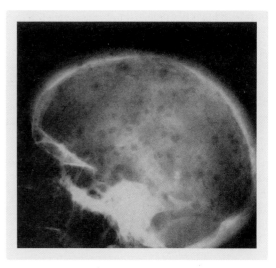

Fig. 5.19 A radiograph of the skull of a patient with multiple myeloma showing many osteolytic bone lesions (courtesy Dr M Makris).

Clinical features

- Bone destruction such as diffuse osteoporosis and pathological fractures are a common feature. They are thought to arise as a result of bone resorption induced by the production of osteoclast-activating factor (OAF) by the myeloma cells. See Fig. 5.19 for the radiographic appearance of multiple myeloma
- Neurological symptoms due to the compression of the spinal cord or roots by collapsed vertebrae
- Normochromic normocytic anaemia results from marrow infiltration
- Repeated infections can occur due to hypogammaglobulinaemia and neutropenia
- Hypercalcaemia occurs in 10% of cases. This is due to increased reabsorption of bone and is indicative of advanced disease
- Chronic renal failure occurs in 20–30% of patients. Factors that can contribute to renal failure in multiple myeloma are:
  - increased blood viscosity
  - hypercalcaemia
  - renal tubular obstruction by proteinaceous casts
  - toxic effect of Bence-Jones protein on proximal renal tubules

  - infection
  - dehydration
  - non-steroidal anti-inflammatory drugs
  - light-chain deposition in glomeruli.
- Amyloidosis (see below) can lead to nephrotic syndrome
- An abnormal bleeding tendency occurs owing to the adverse effect of paraprotein on platelets and coagulation factors.

Solitary myeloma (plasmacytoma)

A plasmacytoma is a solitary tumour found either in the bone or soft tissues, especially the upper respiratory tract. Osseous plasmacytomas usually progress to multiple myeloma. Extraosseous plasmacytomas do not disseminate and, after excision and radiotherapy, prognosis is excellent.

Waldenström's macroglobulinaemia

Waldenström's macroglobulinaemia is a neoplastic monoclonal proliferation of cells derived from the B-cell lineage. A monoclonal IgM paraprotein (macroglobulin) is produced, increasing blood viscosity. Tumour cells are found in blood, bone marrow, lymph nodes and spleen. The incidence is 3–6/100000 a year and is higher in males than in females. Most patients present between the fifth and seventh decade. Survival averages 2–5 years. Bone pain and osteolytic lesions are rare but hyperviscosity syndrome is common. Macroglobulin interferes with platelet function and coagulation factors resulting in a tendency to bleed.

Heavy chain disease

Heavy chain disease is a rare condition where tumour cells secrete incomplete immunoglobulin heavy chain. This is most commonly α heavy chain disease (seen in Mediterranean countries). Heavy chain disease can progress to lymphoma.

Monoclonal gammopathy of undetermined significance

Around 3% of people aged over 65 years have low levels of paraprotein without any symptom of disease. This condition is termed monoclonal gammopathy of uncertain significance (MGUS). There are <10% plasma cells in the marrow, no bone lesions, no anaemia and no renal failure; 10% will progress to myeloma within 10 years.

Amyloidosis

Amyloid is a heterogenous group of proteins, that have a fibrillar ultrastructure resulting in the formation of β-pleated sheets. Examples of amyloid proteins include:

- AA: serum amyloid A (SAA), an acute phase protein
- AL: immunoglobulin light-chain or fragments.

In amyloidosis, amyloid is deposited in tissues. This can be localized or systemic, with renal impairment being a problem. Amyloidosis can occur in the following conditions:

- Chronic inflammatory disease (in which SAA is initially produced as an acute phase response protein)
- Primary disease
- Plasma cell disorders (multiple myeloma, Waldenström's macroglobulinaemia)
- Long-term haemodialysis
- Hereditary (very rare)
- Medullary carcinoma of the thyoid
- Ageing (cardiac or Alzheimer's disease).

Leucopenia

- Leucopenia: reduction in white blood cells, most commonly neutrophils ($<4 \times 10^9$/L).
- Neutropenia (granulocytopenia): reduction in neutrophils ($<1.5 \times 10^9$/L 1 month to 10 years, $<1.8 \times 10^9$/L above 10 years old).
- Agranulocytosis: severe, acute reduction in neutrophils ($<0.5 \times 10^9$/L in peripheral blood). Is associated with risk of infection and can be fatal.
- Lymphopenia: reduction in lymphocyte count ($<1 \times 10^9$/L).

Causes of neutropenia and agranulocytosis

- Inadequate granulopoiesis
- Accelerated removal of granulocytes
- Drug-induced neutropenia.

Inadequate granulopoiesis

Reduced or ineffective production of neutrophils in the bone marrow results in neutropenia. This can be generalized bone marrow failure such as:

- Aplastic anaemia (see p. 96): a group of disorders characterized by anaemia, thrombocytopenia and neutropenia
- Invasion of the bone marrow in leukaemias and lymphomas. Neutropenia is accompanied by anaemia and thrombocytopenia
- Megaloblastic anaemia due to vitamin B_{12} or folate deficiency (see p. 87): this leads to impaired DNA synthesis, resulting in abnormal granulocyte precursors that are more susceptible to destruction
- Chemotherapy
- Myelodysplasia.

Or a specific failure of neutrophil production:

- Congenital (Kostmann's syndrome)
- Exposure to certain drugs (Fig. 5.20)
- Cyclical.

Drugs that can cause neutropenia
Analgesic and anti-inflammatory agents (aminopyrine, phenylbutazone)
Hypnotics and sedatives (clozapine, mianserin, imipramine)
Antimalarials (chloroquine)
Diuretics and antihypertensives [furosemide (frusemide)]
Anticonvulsants (phenytoin, carbamazepine)
Antithyroid drugs (carbimazole)
Antibiotics (chloramphenicol, co-trimoxazole, imipenem)
Hypoglycaemic agents (tolbutamide)
Antirheumatoid drugs (gold, sulfasalazine)

Fig. 5.20 Drugs that can cause neutropenia.

Accelerated removal of granulocytes
- Immune-mediated destruction:
  - idiopathic
  - secondary to other autoimmune diseases, e.g. Felty's syndrome (rheumatoid arthritis associated with leucopenia and splenomegaly)
  - due to drug therapy, e.g. chlorpromazine
  - hypersensitivity and anaphylaxis.
- Hypersplenism causing splenic sequestration of neutrophils
- Severe infection (e.g. typhoid, miliary tuberculosis) resulting in increased peripheral utilization.

Drug-induced neutropenia
Drug-induced neutropenia is increasing in frequency. Two mechanisms operate:

1. Direct toxicity: interference with protein synthesis or cell replication of pluripotent stem cells causes a dose-dependent, generalized bone marrow depression
2. Immune mediated destruction of neutrophils (see drug-induced immune destruction of red cells p. 94): this is not related to drug dose and usually occurs early in the course of the therapy.

Causes of lymphopenia
The causes of lymphopenia are:
- Corticosteroid and other immunosuppressive therapy
- Trauma or surgery
- Cushing's syndrome
- Systemic lupus erythematosus (SLE)
- Hodgkin's lymphoma
- AIDS.

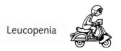

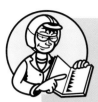

- What cytological features can distinguish between the main types of white blood cell?
- What features of white blood cells are specialized for their function?
- What are the myelodysplastic syndromes and what features are associated with a worse prognosis?
- What is leukaemia and how is it classified?
- What is the Philadelphia chromosome and why is its product a therapeutic target?
- Why does myelofibrosis cause massive splenomegaly?
- What aetiological factors are associated with non-Hodgkin's lymphoma?
- What are the differences between non-Hodgkin's lymphoma and Hodgkin's disease?
- What are the differences between different grades of non-Hodgkin's lymphoma?
- Which cells are pathognomonic of Hodgkin's disease and what is their histological appearance?
- What clinical features are seen in multiple myeloma, and why do they occur?
- What is Bence-Jones protein and why is it seen in multiple myeloma?
- What factors can cause a leucopenia?
- In what conditions is the white-cell count raised?
- Other than myeloma, in which conditions do you get an excess of monoclonal immunoglobulin?
- What are the laboratory features of polycythaemia rubra vera?
- What are leucostatic symptoms and why do they occur in leukaemia?
- What different granules are seen in white blood cells and what do they contain?
- What are common causes of lymphadenopathy?
- How are lymphomas graded and staged?

6. Haemostasis

When a defect such as trauma, inflammation or neoplasia occurs in a vascular wall, bleeding into the vessel wall and surrounding tissues takes place immediately. In normal people, a series of predetermined molecular events (haemostatic response) is initiated.

Haemostatic response: the arrest of bleeding, involving the physiological processes of platelet adhesion, blood coagulation and the contraction of damaged blood vessels.

Three local mechanisms are employed to try to avoid blood loss:
1. Local neurohumoral factors, such as endothelin released by cells adjacent to the injury, induce transient vasoconstriction
2. Primary haemostasis utilizes circulating platelets to form an adhesive plug to slow bleeding
3. Secondary haemostasis (the coagulation cascade) involves circulating plasma proteins. They produce a fibrin network that stabilizes the platelets and traps both red and white blood cells. This stable plug remains until cellular processes repair the damage.

Platelets and blood coagulation

Platelets are disc-shaped, non-nucleated, granule-containing cell fragments with a mean diameter of 2–3 μm (Fig. 6.1). They are formed in the bone marrow from megakaryocyte cytoplasm. The normal lifespan of platelets is 7–10 days and at any time up to a third are sequestered in the spleen.

Platelet structure and production
The normal discoid circulating shape is maintained by a band of 10 to 15 parallel microtubules located around the circumference. Platelets have two tubular

systems: the dense tubular system and the surface-opening canalicular system. Platelets contain three types of granule: α, δ and λ.

Haematopoietic stem cells differentiate to form megakaryoblasts (Fig. 6.2). Megakaryoblasts mature by endomitosis, expanding cytoplasmic volume and increasing the number of nuclear lobes without dividing. This forms a polyploid megakaryocyte, which can produce 2000–7000 platelets. Cytoplasmic processes protrude into sinusoids where they fragment into proplatelets, which then disperse as individual platelets. Platelet production is controlled by:
- Negative feedback: number of circulating platelets
- Thrombopoietin release: increases platelet numbers
- Interleukin-3 (IL-3) and granulocyte–macrophage colony-stimulating factor (GM-CSF)—these stimulate CFU-megakaryocytes (CFU-MK).

Platelet functions
The main functions of platelets are adhesion, release reaction, aggregation, procoagulation and tissue repair.

Adhesion
Normally, endothelial cells have antiplatelet, anticoagulant and fibrinolytic activity. However, as blood oozes through defective vessel wall, platelets become exposed to the extracellular matrix of subendothelial vessel structures. This allow glycoprotein binding and platelet activation. Platelet plasma membrane glycoproteins are essential in mediating platelet interactions with other platelets or subendothelial connective tissue (Fig. 6.3). Examples of glycoprotein (GP) binding are as follows:
- GPIa: binds collagen
- GPIb: binds von Willebrand's factor (vWF). vWF, synthesized by endothelial cells and megakaryocytes, also binds exposed microfibrils
- GPIIb/IIIa: binds either vWF or fibrinogen.

Release reaction
Within 1–2 seconds of adhesion, a monolayer of platelets forms. Platelets change from discs to

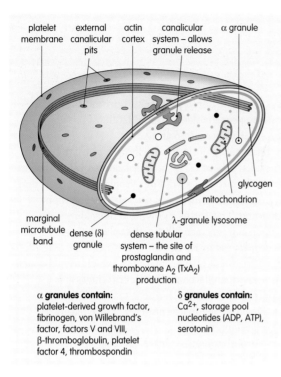

Fig. 6.1 Platelet structure. ADP, adenosine diphosphate; ATP, adenosine triphosphate, Ca²⁺, calcium ions.

α granules contain: platelet-derived growth factor, fibrinogen, von Willebrand's factor, factors V and VIII, β-thromboglobulin, platelet factor 4, thrombospondin

δ granules contain: Ca²⁺, storage pool nucleotides (ADP, ATP), serotonin

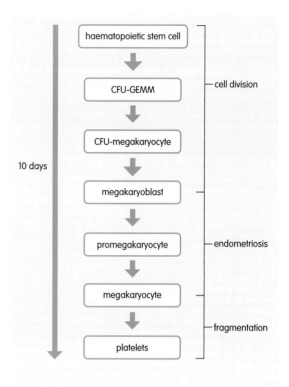

Fig. 6.2 Platelet formation. CFU, colony-forming unit; CFU-GEMM, granulocyte, erythrocyte, monocyte, megakaryocyte colony-forming unit.

spheres with numerous cytoplasmic projections, promoting platelet–platelet interactions. Granule contents are released through the canalicular system.

Platelet aggregation

Granule contents promote further platelet adhesion and aggregation.

1. ADP, from δ granules, alters the surface configuration of locally circulating platelets, which promotes aggregation
2. Subendothelial collagen and thrombin promote ADP release and thromboxane A_2 (TxA_2) production, which potentiate platelet adhesion and aggregation
3. GPIIb/IIIa, exposed on aggregated platelets, binds plasma fibrinogen and promotes aggregation with platelets bound to the subendothelium, vWF and collagen
4. These interactions set up a cycle of further platelet aggregation and release of ADP and TxA_2, resulting in the formation of a platelet plug
5. Thrombin converts fibrinogen to fibrin strengthening the platelet plug.

Prostacyclin (PGI_2), from endothelial cells, inhibits platelet aggregation and interactions with normal endothelium (Fig. 6.4). Aggregation is made irreversible by:

- High levels of ADP
- Platelet-release products
- Platelet contractile proteins.

Procoagulant function

Platelet aggregation rearranges membrane phospholipid (platelet factor III), forming an ideal site for coagulation reactions to take place (see the coagulation pathway, p. 120).

Tissue repair

Platelets stimulate wound healing through platelet-derived growth factor (PDGF), which is mitogenic for vascular smooth muscle cells and fibroblasts.

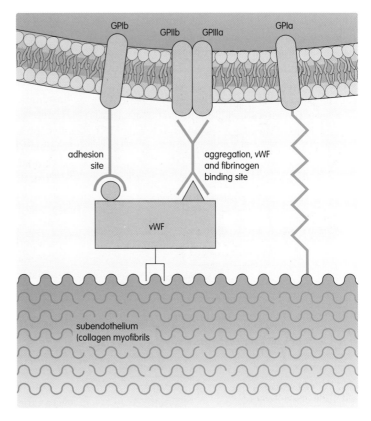

Fig. 6.3 Platelet adhesion reactions. von Willebrand's factor (vWF) binds to damaged vessel walls via subendothelial microfibrils. vWF interacts with platelets via GPIb (calcium required). This leads to exposure of GPIIIb/IIa receptor, which also binds vWF. Platelets bind directly to subendothelial collagen (types I, II and III) via GPIa.

Platelet disorders

The normal concentration of platelets in blood is $150–400 \times 10^9$/L. A reduced platelet count (thrombocytopenia) or defects of platelet function can cause a disorder of bleeding (Fig. 6.5).

Reduced platelet count (thrombocytopenia)
Decreased platelet production
This is the most common cause of thrombocytopenia. The causes are listed in Fig. 6.6.

Generalized disease of the bone marrow
Decreased megakaryocyte production, and therefore platelet production, can be part of a wider clinical picture. Aplastic anaemia is associated with generalized bone marrow failure. Bone marrow infiltration, e.g. due to metastatic carcinoma, also reduces the number of marrow megakaryocytes.

Specific impairment of platelet production
Drugs (thiazide diuretics, ethanol and cytotoxics) can cause thrombocytopenia by several mechanisms:

- Depressing the whole bone marrow
- Specifically impairing megakaryocyte development or proliferation
- Drug-dependent antiplatelet antibody formation (rare).

Viruses can impair platelet production by invading the megakaryocyte, e.g. measles. HIV precipitates the development of antiplatelet antibodies and suppresses megakaryocytes, causing thrombocytopenia in 50% of patients.

Ineffective megakaryopoiesis
Impaired DNA synthesis in megaloblastic anaemia due to vitamin B_{12} or folate deficiency results in ineffective thrombopoiesis.

Decreased platelet survival
The causes of decreased platelet survival are listed in Fig. 6.7.

Immune destruction
Acute ITP is a self-limiting, postviral illness most common in under 10-year-olds. The platelet count is

usually less than $20 \times 10^9/L$. The immune response following an infection such as rubella, chicken pox or measles results in circulation of antibody–viral antigen complexes. The complexes bind to platelets, which are subsequently removed by the reticuloendothelial system. Over 80% of patients recover without treatment, but in 5–10% of cases a chronic form of the disease develops (chronic ITP).

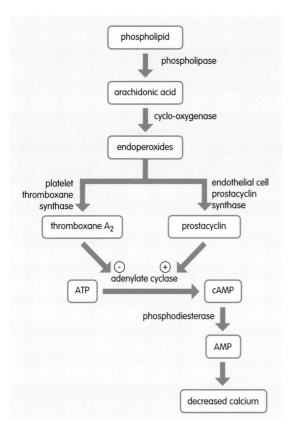

Fig. 6.4 The actions of prostacyclin and thromboxane A_2. AMP, adenosine monophosphate; ATP, adenosine triphosphate; cAMP, cyclic adenosine monophosphate.

Chronic ITP occurs predominantly between the ages of 15 and 50 years. The incidence is greater in women than in men. Patients present with petechiae, ecchymoses, epistaxis and menorrhagia. The platelet count is usually $20–80 \times 10^9/L$. The onset is usually insidious, with no history of a recent viral infection. Platelets are bound by IgG autoantibodies to platelet glycoproteins. The IgG–platelet complexes are removed by splenic macrophages, causing thrombocytopenia. If complement also binds, destruction mainly occurs in the liver. Chronic ITP can be seen in conjunction with disorders causing aberrant immune responses, such as SLE. Chronic ITP rarely resolves spontaneously and is characteristically relapsing and remitting.

Neonatal alloimmune thrombocytopenia is associated with the transfer of antiplatelet antibodies across the placenta, from the mother to the fetus.

Post-transfusion purpura occurs if donor platelets, but not recipient platelets, express the antigen PI^{A1}. Antibodies and thrombocytopenia develop 5–10 days after a transfusion, although the reason for the destruction of the recipient's platelets is unclear.

Drug-induced immune thrombocytopenia occurs via a variety of mechanisms. The platelet count is often less than $10 \times 10^9/L$ and patients present with acute purpura. Drugs known to induce immune thrombocytopenia, e.g. quinine, should be stopped if the patient becomes thrombocytopenia.

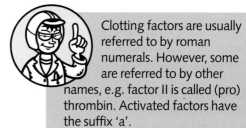

Clotting factors are usually referred to by roman numerals. However, some are referred to by other names, e.g. factor II is called (pro)thrombin. Activated factors have the suffix 'a'.

Fig. 6.5 Platelet count and bleeding tendency.

Platelet count and bleeding tendency	
Platelet count ($\times 10^9/L$)	Bleeding tendency
100–150	Normal haemostasis (if normal function)
20–100	Bleeding time increases: platelet transfusions might be required to cover trauma or surgery
<20	Risk of spontaneous bleeding from skin and mucous membranes and into the brain, pulmonary cavity and retina: prophylactic platelet transfusions to be considered

Non-immune destruction

Thrombotic thrombocytopenic purpura (TTP) is a rare but serious disorder that most commonly affects young adults. It is marked by fever, transient neurological defects and renal failure. Microthrombi (platelets and fibrin) are deposited in arterioles and capillaries, causing thrombocytopenia and microangiopathic haemolytic anaemia (erythrocytes fragment as they circulate through the partially occluded vessels). The exact aetiology of TTP is unknown, but immune-mediated endothelial damage and synthesis of abnormal forms of vWF, causing platelet hyperaggregability, have been proposed as possible contributory factors.

Haemolytic–uraemic syndrome (HUS) is a disorder similar to TTP affecting infants and young children. However, in HUS the platelet–fibrin microthrombi are limited to the kidneys. In many patients, the disease follows recent infections with *Escherichia coli* or other enteric pathogens.

Disseminated intravascular coagulation

See p. 128.

Splenic sequestration

In a normal individual, about 30% of total body platelets are in the spleen at any one time. These are freely exchangeable with those in the circulation. An increase in splenic size (splenomegaly) causes the splenic platelet pool to increase to the point that it may account for up to 90% of total body platelets, resulting in peripheral thrombocytopenia.

Dilutional thrombocytopenia

Whole blood that has been stored for more than 24 hours contains very few viable platelets, owing to their short half-life. Massive transfusion (>10 units/24 hours) of this platelet-poor blood can result in dilutional thrombocytopenia and deficiency of clotting factors II, V and VIII.

Causes of reduced platelet production	
Mechanism	**Cause**
Bone marrow failure	Aplastic anaemia
Bone marrow infiltration	• Metastatic carcinoma • Leukaemia • Lymphoma • Multiple myeloma • Myelofibrosis
Impaired platelet production	• Thiazides • Co-trimoxazole • Phenylbutazone • Alcohol • Chemo- or radiotherapy • Viruses, e.g. measles, HIV
Ineffective megakaryopoiesis	• Megaloblastic anaemia • Myelodysplasia

Fig. 6.6 Causes of reduced platelet production. HIV, human immunodeficiency virus.

Fig. 6.7 Causes of decreased platelet survival. HIV, human immunodeficiency virus.

Causes of decreased platelet survival	
Mechanism	**Cause**
Immune-mediated destruction	• Idiopathic thrombocytopenic purpura • Neonatal alloimmune thrombocytopenia • Post-transfusion purpura • Drugs, e.g. quinine, Rifampicin • Associated with systemic lupus erythematosus, chronic lymphocytic leukaemia or lymphoma
Infections	• Bacterial sepsis, measles, rubella, influenza • HIV • Malaria
Non-immune	• Thrombotic thrombocytopenic purpura • Dilutional loss • Splenomegaly • Disseminated intravascular coagulation

Defects of platelet function

These can be congenital or acquired (Fig. 6.8).

The coagulation cascade

The coagulation pathways

The coagulation pathway (secondary haemostasis) involves a cascade of protein activation leading to the conversion of fibrinogen to fibrin. The proteins involved are known as clotting or coagulation factors. Coagulation can be initiated from within the circulation (intrinsic) or outside the circulation (extrinsic). An overview of the coagulation pathway is shown in Fig. 6.9.

The coagulation cascade is an amplification system that generates thrombin. Thrombin converts fibrinogen into fibrin and therefore stabilizes the clot. The factors required for coagulation are normally found in the circulation as proenzymes or cofactors (Fig. 6.10). The enzymes, except factor XIII, are serine proteases that hydrolyse peptide bonds, amplifying the response. The coagulation factors adhere to activated platelets, e.g. the primary platelet plug. The platelet surface functions as a catalytic membrane for complexes of coagulation factors and is essential for the speed and magnitude of the secondary coagulation response.

The extrinsic pathway

The secondary haemostatic response is initiated by tissue factor (TF), a glycoprotein present on the surface of fibroblasts. The activation of the coagulation cascade by TF is known as the 'extrinsic' pathway because the circulation is not normally exposed to TF. TF forms a complex with factor (F)VIIa, to produce a complex that activates both FX and FIX. FXa is important early in the coagulation cascade. In the presence of the cofactor FVa, FXa activates prothrombin, converting it to thrombin. Thrombin has many functions including:

- Conversion of fibrinogen to fibrin
- Activation of factors V, XI and XIII
- Cleaving FVIII from vWF
- Further platelet activation.

A plasma protein called tissue factor pathway inhibitor (TFPI) binds to and prevents the TF–FVIIa complex activating FX but not FIX. The activation of the cofactor VIII by thrombin allows FIXa to convert FX molecules to FXa. The cofactor V, also activated by thrombin, then aids the formation of more thrombin by FXa. The FIXa/FVIIIa complex is responsible for the continuous FXa formation and subsequent fibrin formation, which is essential for the formation of a durable secondary haemostatic plug.

Prothrombin time (PT) is used to test the extrinsic pathway. Tissue thromboplastin and calcium are added to citrated plasma. A normal clotting time is 10–14 seconds, but the value is normally given as an international normalized ratio (INR).

Activated partial thromboplastin time measures the intrinsic pathway. Phospholipid, a surface activator, and calcium are added to citrated plasma. A normal value is 30–40 seconds.

Causes of defective platelet function		
Type		**Causes**
Congenital	Defective adhesion	Bernard–Soulier syndrome
	Defective aggregation	Glanzmann's thrombasthenia
	Defective secretion	Storage pool diseases
Acquired		Aspirin therapy Uraemia

Fig. 6.8 Causes of defective platelet function.

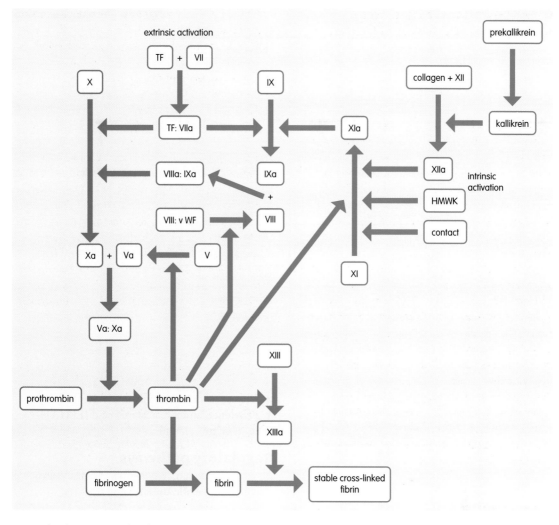

Fig. 6.9 The clotting cascade. The roman numerals indicate the different clotting factors. HMWK, high-molecular-weight kininogen; TF, tissue factor; vWF, von Willebrand's factor.

The intrinsic pathway

The 'intrinsic' pathway begins entirely within the circulation. Reactions between FXII, kallikrein and high-molecular-weight kininogen (HMWK) activate FXI. However, individuals with deficiencies of FXII, kallikrein and HMWK do not exhibit abnormal bleeding. Therefore the physiological role of the intrinsic pathway is uncertain and FXII is not generally considered to be a clotting factor. Intrinsic activation of FXI in major trauma and surgery may be important.

Fibrin

The final step of the secondary coagulation process is the degradation of the plasma protein fibrinogen into small fibrin monomers. These fibrin monomers polymerize spontaneously, by hydrogen bonds, to form long fibres and subsequent complex networks around the primary platelet plug. FXIIIa further stabilizes the clot by forming covalent cross-links between the fibrin polymers.

Role of vitamin K

Factors II, VII, IX and X undergo post-translational γ-carboxylation of glutamic acid residues. The modification of these factors allow them to bind calcium ions and platelet phospholipid membranes. The process, outlined in Fig. 6.11, requires vitamin K as a cofactor. Vitamin K is fat soluble and deficiency is often a result of malabsorption.

121

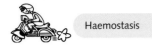

The coagulation factors		
Factor number	**Name**	**Active form**
I	Fibrinogen	Fibrin
II	Prothrombin	Serine Protease
III	Tissue factor (thromboplastin)	Cofactor
V	Labile factor	Cofactor
VII	Proconvertin	Serine Protease
VIII	Antihaemophilic factor	Cofactor
IX	Christmas factor	Serine Protease
X	Stuart–Prower factor	Serine Protease
XI	Plasma thromboplastin antecedent	Serine Protease
XII	Hageman factor	Serine Protease
XIII	Fibrin stabilizing factor	Transglutaminase
Prekallikrein		Serine Protease
High-molecular-weight kininogen (HMWK)		Cofactor

Fig. 6.10 The coagulation factors.

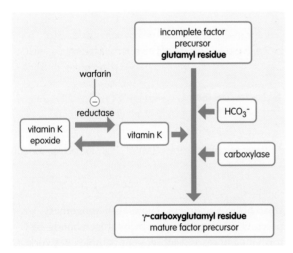

Fig. 6.11 Post-translational modification of the vitamin-K-dependent factors (Factors II, VII, IX, X, proteins C and S). HCO_3^-, bicarbonate ions.

Role of calcium
Adequate levels of calcium are needed to allow clotting, by activating the vitamin-K-dependent factors. Reducing calcium can prevent coagulation of blood samples. This is done by:

- Citrate → deionize calcium
- Ethylenediaminetetraacetic acid (EDTA) → precipitate calcium.

Regulatory pathways
A complex regulatory system prevents extension of coagulation outside the site of injury.

Proteins C and S
Protein C is a serine protease that destroys the activated cofactors Va and VIIIa. It also enhances fibrinolysis by inhibiting tissue plasminogen activator inhibitor (PAI). Protein C is activated when thrombin binds to thrombomodulin on endothelial cells. Protein S is a cofactor for protein C, binding it to the platelet surface (Fig. 6.12). Both proteins C and S are dependent on vitamin K (see Fig. 6.11).

Antithrombin III
Antithrombin III (ATIII) is a potent inhibitor of thrombin, IXa, Xa and XIIa. ATIII binds to the serine residue in the active site of these factors. The inhibitory effect of ATIII is potentiated by heparin.

Anticoagulation
The main use of anticoagulants is to prevent unwanted thrombus formation or extension. They

act on the clotting cascade to prevent fibrin formation. Anticoagulants do not prevent platelet plug formation. There are two commonly used anticoagulants, heparin and warfarin. A table summarizing the attributes of heparin and warfarin is given in Fig. 6.13. The type of anticoagulant and the duration of its use will depend on the indication for treatment. Indications for anticoagulation therapy include:

- Prophylaxis: mechanical prosthetic heart valves, atrial fibrillation, following surgery, unstable angina
- Post-thromboembolic event: deep vein thrombosis, pulmonary embolism, acute peripheral arterial occlusion, management of myocardial infarction
- During therapeutic procedures: cardiopulmonary bypass, haemodialysis.

The danger of using anticoagulants is the risk of haemorrhage. Patients already at risk of bleeding, e.g. those with peptic ulcers, oesophageal varices or severe hypertension, are contraindicated for anticoagulation. People given anticoagulants should be monitored closely to ensure the correct dose is being administered.

Warfarin

Warfarin is a vitamin K antagonist and will therefore reduce the activity of vitamin-K-dependent factors. It affects the factors in the order VII, IX, X and II due to their half-lives. Proteins C and S are also inactivated by warfarin. This occurs before thrombin inactivation causing a relative deficiency in proteins C and S, which can lead to skin necrosis due to extensive thrombosis of the microvasculature within the subcutaneous fat. Because warfarin acts on the extrinsic pathway, the prothrombin time is used to monitor the effect on clotting (given as INR). The target INR for different indications is given in Fig. 6.14.

Care must be taken when using warfarin. It is tetratogenic and therefore should not be used in early pregnancy (heparin does not cross the placenta and so can be used in pregnancy). Warfarin interacts with several drugs. Common interactions are shown in Fig. 6.15. Warfarin is potentiated in liver disease.

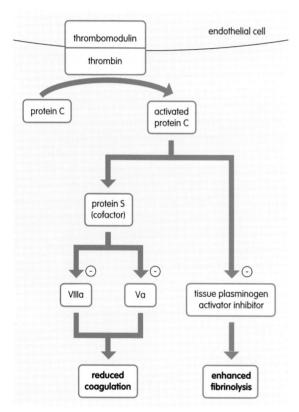

Fig. 6.12 Actions of proteins C and S to limit thrombus formation.

Fig. 6.13 Heparin and warfarin.

Features of heparin and warfarin		
	Heparin (unfractionated)	**Warfarin**
Site of action	Potentiates antithrombin III	Inhibits vitamin K reductase
Route of administration	Subcutaneous/Intravenous	Oral
Prothrombin time	Mildly prolonged	Prolonged
Activated partial thromboplastin time	Prolonged	Prolonged
Thrombin time	Prolonged	Normal

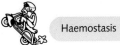

INR for warfarin therapy	
Indication	**Target INR**
DVT prophylaxis	2.5
Treatment of DVT/PE	2.5
Recurrent DVT/PE (on warfarin)	3.5
Atrial fibrillation	2.5
Dilated cardiomyopathy	2.5
Mural thrombus post MI	2.5
Rheumatic mitral valve disease	2.5
Mechanical heart valve	3.5

Fig. 6.14 Target international normalized ratio (INR) for different indications of warfarin therapy. All targets are ±0.5. DVT, deep vein thrombosis; MI, myocardial infarction; PE, pulmonary embolus.

Drug interactions with warfarin	
Increase anticoagulant effect	**Decrease anticoagulant effect**
Sulphonamides	Barbiturates
Metronidazole	Rifampicin
Cephalosporins	Oral contraceptives
Tricyclic antidepressants	Antifungals
Thyroxine	Antiepileptics (e.g.
Amiodarone	carbamazepine)
High-dose salicylates (aspirin)	
Excess paracetamol	
Alcohol	

Fig. 6.15 Common drug interactions with warfarin.

Because warfarin has a half-life of 40 hours, the effects of changes in dose can take 4–5 days to become evident. If there is a warfarin overdose, i.e. the INR exceeds 4.5, warfarin should be stopped for 1 or 2 days and recommenced at a lower dose. The specific antidote to warfarin is vitamin K, which can be administered orally or intravenously. If the overdose has resulted in severe bleeding, fresh-frozen plasma or factor concentrates might be needed.

Heparin

Heparin is a glycosaminoglycan that potentiates the actions of ATIII. Standard (unfractionated) heparin contains molecules ranging in weight from 5000 to 30000kDa. The different chain lengths affect both activity and clearance, with the larger molecules being cleared more quickly. The activated partial thromboplastin time (APTT) is used to monitor unfractionated heparin therapy. Low-molecular-weight heparin (LMWH) has a mean molecular weight of 5000kDa. LMWH is monitored only in renal failure and pregnancy. Monitoring is with an anti-Xa assay. LMWH differs from standard heparin because:

- It has greater activity against factor Xa than thrombin
- It has reduced protein binding and clearance
- Interactions with platelets are reduced.

Heparins are commonly used, as a continuous intravenous infusion, in the acute management of deep vein thrombosis (DVT) and pulmonary embolus (PE). Warfarin therapy is often started within 2 days and heparin stopped when the INR is > 2.0. Intermittent subcutaneous injection, particularly of LMWH is more commonly used. This is the anticoagulant of choice for prophylaxis against venous thrombosis following surgery and is increasingly used as a prophylactic against DVT.

Long-term heparin therapy can result in osteoporosis. Other complications include bleeding and thrombocytopenia. The risk of complications is 50% lower for LMWH than for unfractionated heparin.

Fibrinolysis

In blood, the fibrinolytic system dissolves excessive growth of coagulation products into the lumen of the vessels, thus preventing luminal occlusion. Plasminogen is activated, by cleaving an arginine–valine bond, to form plasmin. Activation can be intrinsic (by FXIIa or kallikrein) or extrinsic (by tissue plasminogen activator (tPA) or urokinase-like A). Many mechanisms, e.g. thrombin-activated fibrinolysis inhibitor, closely regulate fibrinolysis.

Tissue plasminogen activator

tPA is released from activated endothelial cells and is the most important activator of fibrinolysis. It binds to fibrin, where it activates plasminogen that is already bound to the thrombus. This ensures that plasmin production is localized to the clot. Inhibitors of tPA are destroyed by protein C, enhancing fibrinolysis.

Plasmin

Plasmin cleaves peptide bonds in fibrin to produce degradation products of various sizes. Small fragments, termed 'D' fragments, are produced in large quantities in conditions such as disseminated intravascular coagulation (see p. 128). D-dimers can be detected in the plasma or urine using a diagnostic XDP test. The structure of fibrin and the basis for the XDP test are shown in Fig. 6.16. Plasmin also digests:

- Fibrinogen
- Factors V and VIII.

Therapeutic fibrinolysis

Fibrinolytic agents are used in life-threatening venous thrombosis, pulmonary embolism and myocardial infarction. They attempt to restore blood supply to an area of the circulation that has been occluded by a fibrin clot. There are different fibrinolytic agents available:

- Streptokinase: derived from group A β-haemolytic streptococci. It binds to plasminogen to form a complex that can activate other plasminogen molecules. It is highly antigenic
- Urokinase: derived from human kidney cells. It is a tPA originally isolated in urine
- Recombinant tPA: synthesized from human cells. It is highly specific for plasminogen and has a short half-life of 2–6 minutes.

Overview of haemostasis

The role of platelets, the clotting cascade and fibrinolysis in haemostasis are outlined in Fig. 6.17.

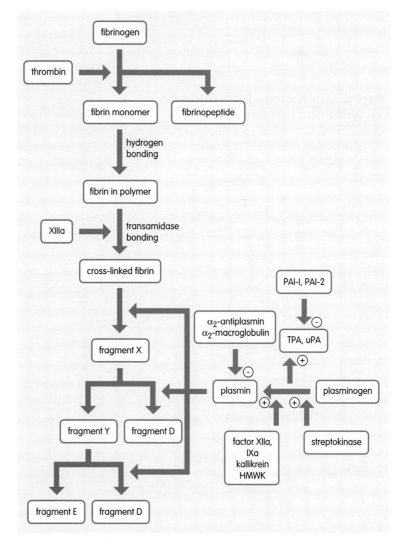

Fig. 6.16 Fibrin and the fibrinolytic system. When plasmin degrades fibrin it produces D fragments, which form dimers. This is the basis for the XDP test, which is used to identify previous clotting, e.g. following deep vein thrombosis. HMWK, high-molecular-weight kininogen; PAI-1 & -2, plasminogen activator inhibitors 1 and 2; tPA, tissue plasminogen activator; uPA, urokinase plasminogen activator.

Haemorrhage: loss of circulating blood.
Petechiae: punctate haemorrhages <2mm in diameter, usually clustered.
Ecchymoses (bruises): diffuse flat haemorrhages under the skin.
Purpura: any condition with bleeding into the skin or mucous membranes.
Haematoma: distinct local swelling caused by loss of blood into muscle or subcutaneous tissue.

hereditary bleeding disorder, affecting 1% of the population. vWF is the carrier protein for factor VIII in plasma, and stabilizes it, prolonging its survival in the circulation. It also promotes platelet interactions. There are several types of the disease:

- Type 1: partial deficiency of circulating vWF
- Type 2A: absence of the largest vWF subunits
- Type 2B: synthesis of abnormal vWF multimers
- Type 2M: defective GP1b binding site
- Type 2N: reduced affinity for factor VIII
- Type 3: absolute deficiency of circulating vWF.

Type 1 is the most common form of the disease. Impaired release of normally synthesized vWF multimers from endothelial cells leads to a deficiency of vWF. This can be partially corrected by an infusion of arginine vasopressin.

The severity of clinical symptoms is very variable. The impairment of platelet adhesion and factor VIII deficiency can cause mucous membrane bleeding and excessive blood loss following injuries and surgery. In type 3 disease there may be spontaneous bleeds into muscles and joints.

Clotting factor disorders

Clotting factor abnormalities can be hereditary or acquired.

Hereditary factor abnormalities
von Willebrand's disease
von Willebrand's disease, a deficiency or defect in von Willebrand's factor (vWF) is the most common

Haemophilia A
Haemophilia A is caused by a deficiency of factor VIII. The prevalence of haemophilia A in males is 1

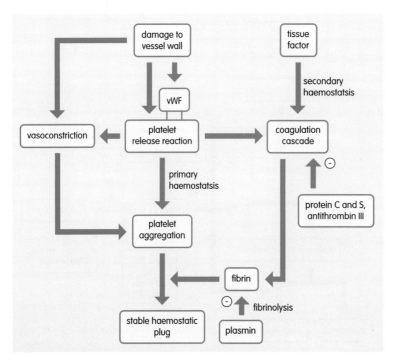

Fig. 6.17 Overview of haemostasis. vWF, von Willebrand's factor.

in 5000 and is not affected by geographic, ethnic or religious association, or by social class. Haemophilia A is an X-linked recessive condition, therefore overwhelmingly affecting males. In 33% of all haemophilia A cases, patients have no family history of the disease and such cases are thought to arise from spontaneous mutation of the factor VIII gene. The normal plasma concentration of factor VIII ranges from 0.5 to 2IU/mL. The frequency and severity of bleeding correlates with the plasma level of factor VIII. Haemophilia A can be classified as severe, moderate or mild (Fig. 6.18) with severe disease accounting for ~70% of haemophilic patients.

Common sites of bleeding
- Haemarthroses: joint bleeding episodes are usually located in the weight bearing joints
- Haematomas: muscular bleeding episodes are typically located in the extremities
- Central nervous system often traumatic, epi- or subdural haemorrhage
- Ear, nose and throat.

Some of the most serious consequences of bleeds include:
- Chronic damage: fixed flexion deformities of the limbs with muscle atrophy, hearing impairment, neurological damage
- Acute problems: compartment syndrome, compression of the respiratory tract, massive loss of circulating volume.

Factor replacement therapy
Factor VIII can be replaced with:
- Fresh-frozen plasma
- Cryoprecipitate
- Factor VIII concentrates
- Recombinant factor VIII.

These can be infused following injury to raise the level of factor VIII to between 30 and 100% of normal. Prophylactic treatment with factor VIII is currently recommended in children with severe haemophilia. The baseline of FVIII is raised above 2%, converting 'severe' to 'moderate' disease.

There is a risk of iatrogenic infections from all blood products. Haemophiliacs are exposed to blood products from many donors (pooled plasma is used to concentrate factor VIII) on many occasions each year (average 31 bleeding episodes per year). Over 50% of haemophiliacs in the USA and Europe contracted HIV from blood products before screening for HIV was introduced; many also contracted hepatitis C. AIDS has been a common cause of death in haemophiliacs, with many also developing chronic hepatitis and cirrhosis.

Haemophilia B
Haemophilia B (Christmas disease), caused by a deficiency of factor IX, is also X-linked. Haemophilia A and B can be differentiated only by specific coagulation factor assays. Haemophilia B has an identical pattern of clinical features to haemophilia A, but is five times less common. Treatment is similar to that for haemophilia A, but with factor IX replacement rather than VIII. Factor IX has a longer

Fig. 6.18 Haemophilia symptoms.

Symptoms of haemophilia A	
Concentration of coagulation factor (% of normal)	**Bleeding episodes**
50–100	None
25–50	Bleeding tendency after severe trauma
5–25 Mild	Severe bleeding episodes after surgery, slight bleeding episodes after minor trauma
1–5 Moderate	Severe bleeding episodes even after slight trauma
<1 Severe	Spontaneous bleeding episodes predominantly in the joints or muscles

half-life than factor VIII and therefore fewer infusions are required.

Other deficiencies

Hereditary deficiencies of the other coagulation factors are rare. As in haemophilias A and B, the severity of the disorders is related to the degree of deficiency. In specific areas, the prevalence of a certain coagulation factor deficiency can be much higher than average. Examples of this are a high prevalence of FVII deficiency in Northern Italy and a high prevalence of FXI deficiency among Ashkenazi Jews.

Figure 6.19 shows a summary of hereditary factor deficiencies.

Acquired factor abnormalities
Vitamin K deficiency

Vitamin K deficiency was discussed on page 121.

Liver disease

The liver produces all the clotting factors except for vWF; liver disease is therefore associated with clotting factor deficiency. In addition, biliary obstruction can lead to malabsorption and deficiency of fat-soluble vitamin K. This leads to decreased synthesis of the vitamin-K-dependent factors. Portal hypertension can lead to splenomegaly, resulting in increased splenic sequestration of platelets. In severe liver disease, levels of factor V and fibrinogen are reduced, and increased levels of plasminogen activator are present. An acquired dysfibrinogenaemia (functional abnormality of fibrinogen) is also seen in many patients.

Disseminated intravascular coagulation (DIC)

DIC arises from excessive activation of the coagulation cascade, followed by activation of the fibrinolytic system. Coagulation is activated in two ways:
1. Release of tissue factor from damaged tissues, monocytes or red blood cells
2. Activation of factors XII and XI by damaged vascular endothelium.

There is generalized fibrin deposition on vascular endothelium, with extensive consumption of platelets and coagulation factors. Small vessels are obstructed, leading to tissue damage and multiple organ dysfunction.

Fibrin deposition activates the fibrinolytic pathway and results in the formation of fibrin degradation products (FDPs). FDPs inhibit fibrin polymerization and consequently impair coagulation. The net result is a bleeding disorder due to a lack of platelets and clotting factors and inhibition of fibrin polymerization by FDPs. In DIC, PT, APTT and thrombin clotting times can all be prolonged.

Overview of hereditary clotting factor abnormalities			
Feature	Haemophilia A	Haemophilia B	von Willebrand's disease
Deficiency	Factor VIII	Factor IX	vWF and moderate reduction in factor VIII
Inheritance	X-linked	X-linked	Autosomal dominant with incomplete penetration
Main sites of bleeding	Muscles, joints, post-trauma/surgery	Muscles, joints, post-trauma/surgery	Mucous membranes, skin cuts, post-trauma/surgery
Platelet count	Normal	Normal	Normal
Platelet aggregation	Normal	Normal	Impaired
Bleeding time	Normal	Normal	Prolonged
Prothrombin time	Normal	Normal	Normal
APTT	Prolonged	Prolonged	Prolonged or normal

Fig. 6.19 Overview of the major hereditary clotting factor deficiencies. APTT, activated partial thromboplastin time; vWF, von Willebrand's factor.

Causes of DIC include:
- Acute: obstetric complications, septicaemia, acute haemolysis, shock
- Subacute: malignancy
- Chronic: liver disease, malignancy, eclampsia.

The management of DIC involves treatment of the underlying disorder and supportive care with transfusion of fresh frozen plasma, cryoprecipitate and platelets. Heparin can be used in low-grade DIC to prevent microthrombi formation, although it might exacerbate bleeding.

Thrombosis

 Thrombosis is the formation of a blood clot (thrombus) in the circulation from blood constituents.

Virchow's triad

Virchow's triad outlines the factors that predispose to thrombus formation:
- Changes in blood flow
- Changes in blood constituents
- Changes within the walls of blood vessels.

Hypercoagulability

Thrombophilias are disorders of haemostasis that increase the tendency of blood to clot. These may be inherited or acquired.

Primary (hereditary) thrombophilia
Antithrombin III deficiency

ATIII deficiency is an autosomal dominant condition affecting 1 in 2000 people. The deficiency is either:
- Type I (decreased quantity)
- Type II (reduced biological activity).

Heterozygotes have 40–50% of normal plasma ATIII levels; homozygosity is lethal. Most patients with ATIII deficiency experience a thrombotic episode before the age of 50 years. Thrombosis might be severe and recurrent and these patients might have to have their blood anticoagulated with oral warfarin (see also p. 123).

Deficiencies of proteins C and S

Inheritance for both protein C and protein S deficiencies is autosomal dominant. Protein S deficiency is clinically indistinguishable from protein C deficiency (see also p. 122). As with ATIII deficiency, they can be type I (decreased quantity) or type II (reduced biological activity). Heterozygotes have 50% of normal levels of proteins C or S and clinical features are similar to ATIII deficiency, but the thrombotic risk is four times lower. Homozygous individuals have less than 1% of normal levels of proteins C or S. Because proteins C and S have a shorter half-life than vitamin-K-dependent factors II, IX and X, warfarin therapy causes a prothrombotic state and can lead to skin necrosis.

Defective fibrinolysis

Abnormal plasminogen and fibrinogen have been associated with reduced fibrinolytic activity and a tendency of blood to clot.

Activated protein C resistance due to factor V Leiden

A missense mutation of the factor V gene (arginine is replaced by glutamine) renders factor V ten times less sensitive to inactivation by activated protein C. This disorder has an incidence in Caucasians of 5% and it might account for the majority of cases of inherited thrombophilia. This mutation acts as a cofactor in the following hypercoagulable states:
- Oral contraceptive pill and pregnancy
- Surgery and immobility
- Other thrombophilia disorders.

Prothrombin allele G20210A

Two to three per cent of the population have this prothrombin variant, which increases prothrombin levels and the thrombotic risk.

Hyperhomocysteinaemia

High levels of plasma homocysteine increase the risk of venous and arterial thrombosis.

Secondary (acquired) thrombophilia

The following conditions are associated with an increased incidence of thrombosis:

- Prolonged immobilization of the patient (venous stasis)
- Disseminated cancer (secretion of tumour substances that activate factor X)
- Oestrogen therapy (increased plasma levels of factors II, VII, IX and X, and reduced levels of ATIII and tPA)
- Myeloproliferative disorders
- Sickle-cell anaemia
- The antiphospholipid antibody syndrome (lupus anticoagulant syndrome). This disorder is characterized by the presence of antiphospholipid antibodies. The main features of this syndrome are arterial and venous thrombosis in renal, cerebral and mesenteric vessels. The disease can be idiopathic or secondary to other autoimmune disorders such as SLE.

Endothelial injury
Factors such as smoking, hypercholesterolaemia, hypertension, infection and immune-mediated damage, contribute to endothelial injury and subsequent thrombus formation.

Alterations to blood flow
In conditions such as atrial fibrillation, where the flow of blood is altered, thrombus can form within the circulation.

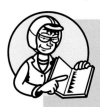

- What mechanisms operate to avoid blood loss following trauma?
- Outline the formation of platelets.
- Explain how platelet aggregation occurs.
- What are the actions of prostacyclin and thromboxane A_2 in the platelet, and how do they affect platelet function?
- List the causes of decreased platelet survival.
- What are the consequences of thrombocytopenia?
- Highlight the differences between the extrinsic and intrinsic pathways of coagulation and the effects of defects in either pathway on standard laboratory coagulation tests.
- The coagulation cascade is an amplification system, what does this mean and why is it important for clotting?
- Why is vitamin K required for clotting?
- What physiological mechanisms regulate coagulation?
- How do heparin and warfarin reduce coagulation?
- When is anticoagulant therapy used?
- What is von Willebrand's disease and what is the clinical presentation?
- Highlight the differences and similarities between haemophilia A and B.
- How are haemophilia A and B treated and what are the risks involved in this treatment?
- Why does liver disease lead to decreased coagulation?
- What causes disseminated intravascular coagulation and what laboratory findings would you expect?
- How does factor V Leiden cause a hypercoagulable state?
- What is Virchow's triad?
- What fibrinolytic agents are available and when should they be used?

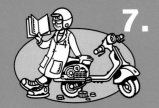

7. Haematological Investigations

Full blood count and reticulocyte count

Blood samples are added to EDTA, an anticoagulant. The samples are tested by an automated analyser, which provides the following information:
- Hb concentration, haematocrit, red-cell count, mean cell volume (MCV) and mean cell haemoglobin (MCH)
- White-cell count with differential
- Platelet count.

Red-cell parameters and the diagnostic inferences of abnormalities of the full blood count are shown in Fig. 7.1.

Differential white count

The differential white count breaks down the white-cell count to identify the level of each of the five peripheral white cell lines; neutrophils, lymphocytes, monocytes, eosinophils and basophils. This is automated and uses stains, cell size and light scatter to differentiate between the different cells. The parameters for white cells and platelets, and the diagnostic inferences made from their abnormalities, are given in Fig. 7.2.

Peripheral blood film

Examination of a peripheral blood film is a simple haematological investigation, which can provide a significant amount of information. Blood is evenly spread into a film on a glass slide, which is then dried and stained, most often with a Romanowsky stain. The peripheral blood film shows the morphology of blood cells and can show inclusions within the cells. Abnormalities of red and white cells that are identified on the peripheral blood film are shown in Figs 7.3 and 7.4 respectively.

Normal blood cells

Normal peripheral blood films are shown in Figs 7.5–7.11.
Peripheral blood films can be used in the diagnosis of haematological disease, for example:
- Iron-deficiency anaemia (Fig. 7.12)
- Hereditary spherocytosis (Fig. 7.13)
- Sickle-cell anaemia (Fig. 7.14)
- Multiple myeloma (Fig. 7.15).

The concept of right shift is illustrated in Fig. 7.16.

Investigations of haemoglobinopathies

Electrophoresis
This is used in the diagnosis of haemoglobinopathies (Fig. 7.17) and the thalassaemia syndromes.

Bone marrow investigation

Bone marrow smear
Bone marrow smears allow examination of the stages of haemopoiesis. Bone marrow smears are usually stained with Romanowsky dyes, but Perls' Prussian blue may be used to detect iron in macrophages and erythroblasts. Fig. 7.18 shows a normal bone marrow smear.

Collection of bone marrow
- Aspiration of bone marrow involves the insertion of a hollow needle into the sternum or iliac crest. Individual cell detail can be assessed from aspirates
- Trephine biopsy involves insertion of a large-bore needle into the iliac crest. A core of bone and marrow is obtained, which is examined as a histological specimen. These specimens are useful for assessing marrow architecture and cellularity.

The bone marrow findings in some disorders are listed in Fig. 7.19.

Red-cell parameters on peripheral full blood count			
Parameter	Normal range		Diagnostic inference of abnormalities
	Male	Female	
Red-cell count	$4.4–5.8 \times 10^{12}$/L	$4.0–5.2 \times 10^{12}$/L	
Haemoglobin	13–17g/dL	12–15g/dL	↑ Polycythaemia ↓ Anaemia
Packed cell volume or Haematocrit	40–51%	38–48%	
Mean cell volume	80–100fL		↑ (macrocytic) Vitamin B$_{12}$ or folate deficiency, pregnancy, neonates, alcohol or chronic liver disease (may be haemolysis or aplastic anaemia) ↓ (microcytic) iron deficiency, thalassaemia or anaemia of chronic disease
Mean cell haemoglobin	27–32pg		↓ (hypochromic) Occurs with microcytosis
Mean cell haemoglobin concentration	32–36g/dL		
Reticulocyte count	1–2% of circulating red cells $10–100 \times 10^9$/L		↑ (Reticulocytosis) haemolytic anaemias and after acute blood loss ↓ (reticulocytopenia) Impaired red-cell production

Fig. 7.1 Red-cell parameters on peripheral full blood count. Packed cell volume otherwise known as the haematocrit is equal to the red-cell count multiplied by the mean cell volume. Mean cell haemoglobin is the haemoglobin divided by the red-cell count, while the mean cell haemoglobin concentration is the haemoglobin divided by the haematocrit. Automated analysers are increasingly able to carry out reticulocyte counts, although they are also carried out on peripheral blood films stained with new methylene blue. The normal range represents values for 95% of the population (mean ±2 standard deviations).

The differential white count		
Parameters	Normal range	Diagnostic inference
White cell count	$4–11 \times 10^9$/L	↑ (leucocytosis); ↓ (leucopenia)
Neutrophils	$2–7.5 \times 10^9$/L (40–80%)	↑ (neutrophilia); ↓ (neutropenia)
Lymphocytes	$1.3–3.5 \times 10^9$/L (20–40%)	↑ (lymphocytosis); ↓ (lymphopenia)
Monocytes	$0.2–0.8 \times 10^9$/L (2–10%)	↑ (monocytosis)
Eosinophils	$0.04–0.44 \times 10^9$/L (1–6%)	↑ (eosinophilia)
Basophils	$0–0.1 \times 10^9$/L (<1–2%)	↑ (basophilia)
Platelet count	$150–400 \times 10^9$/L	↑ Reactive (thrombocytosis): haemorrhage, infection, malignancy, inflammation; or pathological (thrombocythaemia); myeloproliferative disorders ↓ (thrombocytopenia)

Fig. 7.2 The differential white-cell count and its abnormalities. Percentages given indicate the normal percentage of the white-cell count. Abnormalities of white cells can be seen in Chapter 5, thrombocytopenia is covered in Chapter 6. The normal range represents values for 95% of the population (mean ±2 standard deviations).

Red cell abnormalities on the peripheral blood film

Abnormality	Description	Diagnostic inferences
Anisocytosis	Increased variation in size	See causes of micro- and macrocytosis in Fig. 7.1
Poikilocytosis	Increased variation in shape	Certain shapes are diagnostic for certain conditions
Spherocytes	Small spherical cells lacking central pallor	Hereditary spherocytosis, warm AIHA
Sickle cells	Crescent-shaped cells	Sickle-cell anaemia
Target cells	Cells with central and peripheral dark-staining areas separated by a clear area	Thalassaemia syndromes, sickle-cell syndromes, iron deficiency, liver disease
Teardrop cells	Teardrop-shaped cells	Myelofibrosis, extramedullary haemopoiesis
Elliptocyte	Elliptical cell	Hereditary elliptocytosis
Echinocyte	Long projections from cell surface	Renal disease
Acanthocyte	Irregular outline	Liver disease, post-splenectomy, abetalipoproteinaemia
Fragments	Small red cell fragments	DIC, Microangiopathy, cardiac valve replacement
Howell–Jolly bodies	Small nuclear inclusions normally removed by the spleen	Postsplenectomy, hyposplenism
Heinz bodies	Precipitates of oxidized denatured haemoglobin	Glucose-6-phosphate dehydrogenase deficiency
Hypochromia	Large area of central pallor	Reduced mean cell haemoglobin (see Fig. 7.1)
Reticulocytosis (polychromasia)	Large, bluish cells best seen on supravital staining with new methylene blue	See Fig. 7.1
Rouleaux	Red cell stacking	Multiple myeloma, Waldenstrom's macroglobulinaemia

Fig. 7.3 Red cell abnormalities on the peripheral blood film. The normal red cell is normochromic, normocytic and has an area of central pallor. AIHA, autoimmune haemolytic anaemia; DIC, disseminated intravascular coagulation.

White cell abnormalities on the peripheral blood film

Abnormality	Description	Diagnostic inferences
Hypersegmented neutrophils	Neutrophil nucleus containing >5 lobes	Megaloblastic anaemia
Left shift of myeloid cells	Immature myeloid cells, e.g. band cells, metamyelocytes	Pregnancy, severe infection, chronic myeloid leukaemia
Blast cells	Variable appearance	Acute myeloblastic or lymphoblastic leukaemia
Auer rods	Rod-like inclusions within the cytoplasm of leukaemic blasts and promyelocytes	Acute myeloblastic leukaemia
Smear cells	'Smudges' representing disrupted cells	Lymphocytosis—usually chronic lymphocytic leukaemia, but not always malignant
Leucoerythroblastic change	Nucleated red cells and immature leucocytes	Severe haemorrhage/haemolysis, bone marrow infiltration

Fig. 7.4 White cell abnormalities on the peripheral blood film.

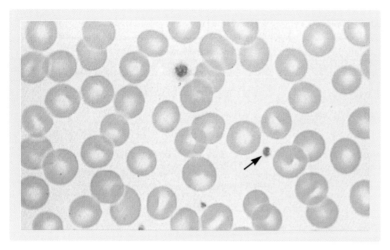

Fig. 7.5 Normal red cells and platelets. Normal red cells are ~7.2 μm in diameter, and have a central pallor due to their biconcave shape. Platelets are seen on the film as small, irregular, densely staining cells (courtesy Professor Victor Hoffbrand and Dr John Pettit).

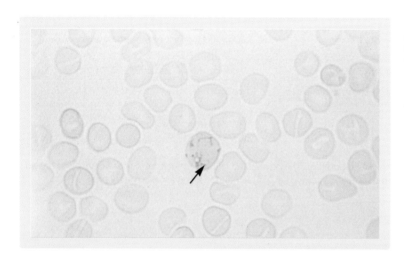

Fig. 7.6 Reticulocytes can be detected using supravital staining, which precipitates RNA in the cell. They are usually present in the blood in small numbers (courtesy Professor Victor Hoffbrand and Dr John Pettit).

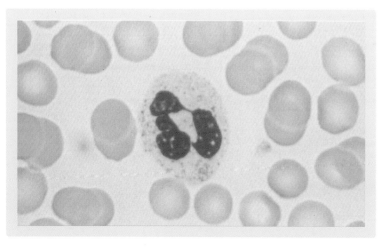

Fig. 7.7 Normal neutrophils have a characteristic multilobed nucleus (connected by chromatin). The cytoplasm is granular (courtesy Professor Victor Hoffbrand and Dr John Pettit).

Fig. 7.8 Normal eosinophils are usually slightly larger than neutrophils. They have a bilobed nucleus and coarse granules (courtesy Professor Victor Hoffbrand and Dr John Pettit).

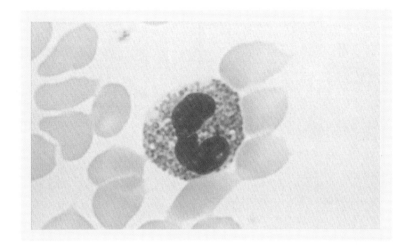

Fig. 7.9 Normal basophils contain a lobed nucleus with very coarse granules. They are the least common white cell in the blood (courtesy Professor Victor Hoffbrand and Dr John Pettit).

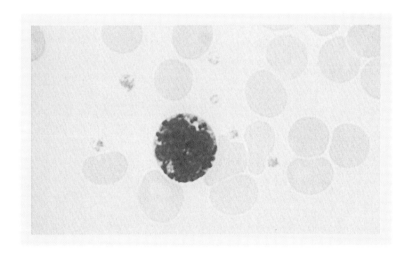

Fig. 7.10 Normal monocytes are large. The nucleus tends to be folded not lobed, and the cytoplasm contains very fine granules (courtesy Professor Victor Hoffbrand and Dr John Pettit).

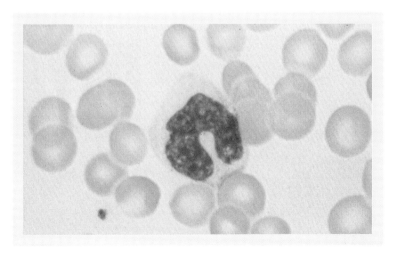

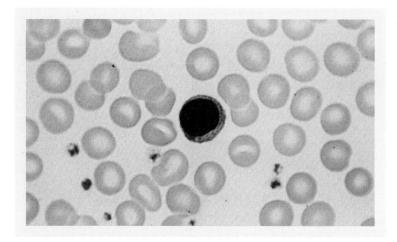

Fig. 7.11 Normal lymphocytes are quite small (9μm diameter). They contain very little cytoplasm and occasional azurophilic granules (courtesy Professor Victor Hoffbrand and Dr John Pettit).

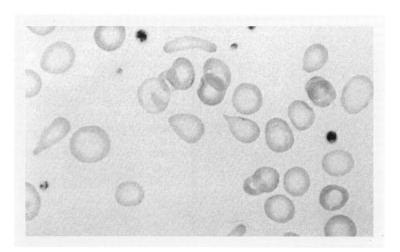

Fig. 7.12 Iron-deficiency anaemia. Red blood cells are typically hypochromic and microcytic (courtesy Professor Victor Hoffbrand and Dr John Pettit).

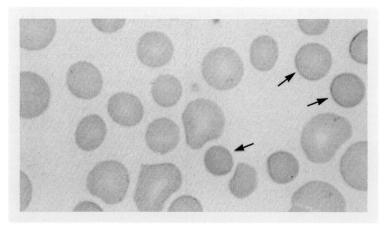

Fig. 7.13 Hereditary spherocytosis. Spherocytes are smaller and thicker than normal red cells but only totally spherical in extreme cases (courtesy Professor Victor Hoffbrand and Dr John Pettit).

Fig. 7.14 Sickle-cell anaemia. Sickled cells are variable in shape, but classically are crescentric. Target cells are also commonly seen (courtesy Professor Victor Hoffbrand and Dr John Pettit).

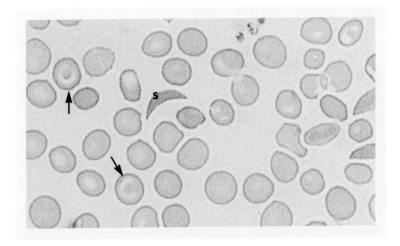

Fig. 7.15 Multiple myeloma. Red cell rouleaux (stacked cells) are seen due to the excess high-molecular-weight proteins in the blood (courtesy Professor Victor Hoffbrand and Dr John Pettit).

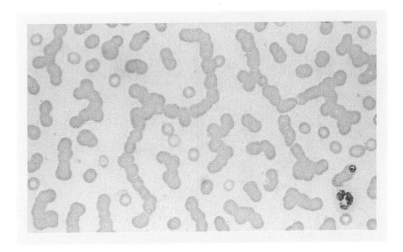

Fig. 7.16 Right shift. Using a neutrophil with a three-lobed nucleus as a marker for normal granulocyte maturation, a shift of development to either the right or left can be seen. Hypermature neutrophils (right shift) are seen in non-infections inflammatory processes, e.g. malignancy, megaloblastic anaemia, iron deficiency, liver disease, uraemia. Left shift is seen by the presence of immature 'band' forms. This occurs due to neutrophil leucocytosis, in this example left shift is due to abdominal sepsis (courtesy Professor Victor Hoffbrand and Dr John Pettit).

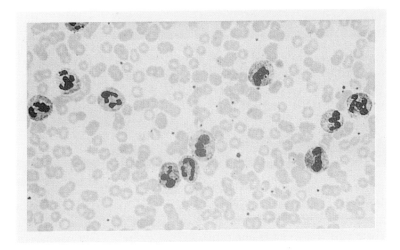

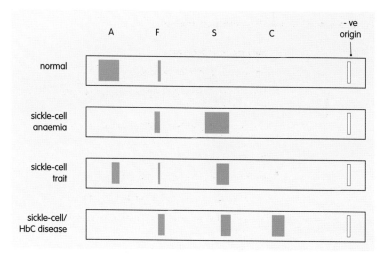

Fig. 7.17 Haemoglobin electrophoresis is used to detect different forms of haemoglobin (Hb). It can detect HbS (sickle haemoglobin), HbC, HbF (fetal haemoglobin), HbA (adult haemoglobin) and HbH (β tetramer sometimes represented as β_4). Note that HbA is greater than HbS in sickle-cell trait.

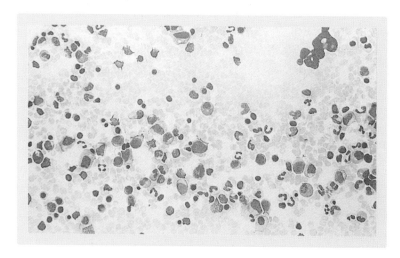

Fig. 7.18 Normal bone marrow smear. Haemopoietic cells and supporting reticuloendothelial cells are usually seen (courtesy Professor Victor Hoffbrand and Dr John Pettit).

Lymph node biopsy

Lymph nodes are biopsied for histological examination when malignancy is suspected. A lymph node biopsy from a patient with Hodgkin's lymphoma is shown in Fig. 7.20.

Cytogenetic analysis

Cytogenetic analysis is the study of structure and function of chromosomes. Certain cytogenetic abnormalities are strongly associated with specific conditions. Important examples in haematology are:

- t(9;22): this is found in chronic myeloid leukaemia (the altered chromosome 22 is called the Philadelphia chromosome)
- t(14;18): this is associated with follicle centre lymphomas
- t(8;14): this is associated with Burkitt's lymphoma.

ESR and plasma viscosity

The erythrocyte sedimentation rate (ESR) is the rate of fall of a column of red cells in plasma over 1 hour. The normal range in men is 1–5mm/hour and in

Appearance of the bone marrow in some haematological disorders	
Disorder	**Bone marrow appearance**
Iron-deficiency anaemia	Absent iron stores from macrophages
Megaloblastic anaemia	Hypercellular marrow with megaloblasts present; giant metamyelocytes often seen
Haemolytic anaemia	Hypercellular marrow with erythroid hyperplasia; reduced myeloid/erythroid ratio (usually 2–8)
Aplastic anaemia	Hypocellular marrow
Acute leukaemia	Hypercellular marrow infiltrated with blasts
Chronic lymphocytic leukaemia	Hypercellular marrow with lymphocytic infiltration
Chronic myeloid leukaemia	Hypercellular marrow with granulocytic and megakaryocytic hyperplasia
Multiple myeloma	Increased proportion of plasma cells (often abnormal)
Polycythaemia rubra vera and essential thrombocythaemia	Hypercellular marrow with hyperplasia of all cell lineages
Myelofibrosis	Early—hypercellularity, late—reactive fibrosis of the bone marrow and reduced haemopoiesis

Fig. 7.19 Appearance of the bone marrow in some haematological disorders (courtesy Professor Victor Hoffbrand and Dr John Pettit).

Fig. 7.20 Hodgkin's lymphoma on lymph node biopsy showing two binucleate Reed—Sternberg cells (arrows). Demonstration of Reed—Sternberg cells (or variants) against a background of inflammatory cells is required to diagnose Hodgkin's lymphoma.

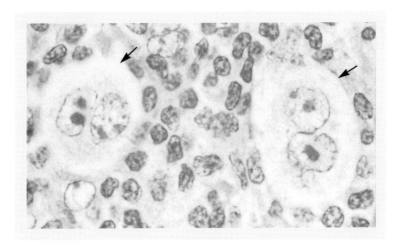

women 5–15mm/hour. ESR is raised with increased plasma viscosity, which is a more easily automated test. The concentration of proteins (fibrinogen and globulins) in the plasma is the major determinant of viscosity. ESR and plasma viscosity are used as indicators of the acute phase response. ESR is raised in inflammation (including response to infection), malignancy (including myeloma) and anaemia. The ESR of pregnant women also increases.

Serum electrophoresis

Normal serum proteins

Proteins in the plasma are vital to maintain colloid osmotic pressure and circulating volume (albumin), to respond to infectious challenges (globulins), for haemostasis (clotting factors) and for transport (e.g. transferrin). These proteins can be distinguished by electrophoresis to produce several bands including:

Tests of the coagulation cascade		
Text	**Normal range**	**Causes of abnormalities**
Thrombin time	10–12 seconds	Heparin therapy DIC Afibrinogenaemia
Prothrombin time	12–14 seconds	Deficiencies of factors II, V, VII and X Liver disease Warfarin therapy DIC
Activated partial thromboplastin time	30–40 seconds	Deficiencies of factors II, V, VIII, IX, X, XI, XII von Willebrand's disease DIC Heparin therapy

Fig. 7.21 Tests of the coagulation cascade. (DIC, disseminated intravascular coagulation).

- Albumin
- α_1-antitrypsin
- α_2-macroglobulin, haptoglobin
- β-transferrin
- γ-globulins.

Acute phase proteins

Following a variety of insults, the liver synthesizes increased quantities of proteins. These proteins, normally present in serum in small amounts, include:

- α_1-antitrypsin
- Fibrinogen
- Complement
- Haptoglobin
- C-reactive protein.

ESR and plasma viscosity indirectly measure the acute phase response by detecting changes in the 'thickness' of plasma. C-reactive protein (CRP) can be measured directly. CRP changes more rapidly than ESR (it will fall within 2–3 days of recovery), so is more sensitive to changes in the response to therapy or in disease activity. Unlike ESR, CRP is not raised in pregnancy or anaemia.

Clotting tests

Prothrombin time (PT), activated partial thromboplastin time and thrombin time are tests of the function of the coagulation cascade. A summary of their normal range and causes of abnormal results are shown in Fig. 7.21.

Specific factor assays can be used to identify deficiencies of single coagulation factors. This is of relevance to haemophilia when an assay can indicate the level of factor in the blood and therefore severity of disease.

Fibrinogen degradation products are used to identify clots, e.g. post-DVT/disseminated intravascular coagulation. These clotting tests are discussed in Chapter 6.

8. Blood Transfusion

Red-cell antigens

The surfaces of red cells are covered with antigenic molecules. Over 400 different groups of antigens have been identified, although only some of these are clinically important in blood transfusion. Some red-cell antigens can be recognized by antibodies in the serum of a recipient of a blood transfusion, and can cause an adverse reaction. These reactions can be severe and life threatening, so it is important to identify the antigens and antibodies present in both donor and recipient blood.

ABO antigens

The ABO system consists of three allelic genes, A, B and O, which code for sugar-residue transferase enzymes. The ABO antigen, known as the H antigen, is a glycoprotein or glycolipid with a terminal L-fructose.

- The O gene is amorphous, i.e. it has no effect on antigenic structure and leaves antigen H unchanged
- The group A gene-product adds N-acetyl galactosamine to the H antigen
- The group B gene-product adds the sugar D-galactose (Fig. 8.1).

Inheritance of the three ABO alleles can lead to six different genotypes and four possible phenotypes (Fig. 8.2).

By 6 months of age, the immune system will have been exposed to A- and B-like antigens in intestinal bacteria and food substances. IgM antibodies develop against A and/or B antigens, unless these antigens are present on red cells. Transfused blood must be ABO-compatible with the recipient's blood, otherwise recipient antibody will cause agglutination and haemolysis of the transfused cells. For example, if group A red cells are given to a group O recipient, anti-A antibodies in the recipient's serum will destroy the donor cells.

Ideally, ABO-identical blood is used, however if this is not possible, compatible blood can be used. Blood cells of group O are not affected by anti-A or anti-B antibodies and can therefore be given to patients of any blood group. Consequently, blood group O is referred to as the universal donor. Conversely, AB individuals are universal recipients because they do not possess anti-ABO antibodies and can receive blood of any ABO type.

Rhesus antigens

Rhesus (Rh) antigens are good immunogens and the antibodies generated are clinically important. They are known as C, D and E, but the D antigen is the most important clinically; it is the D antigen that is referred to when describing someone as 'rhesus positive' or 'rhesus negative'. The rhesus locus on chromosome 1 consists of two closely linked genes, RhD and RhCE, which are inherited together. RhD encodes the D antigen; 'd' denotes the absence of D antigen (Fig. 8.3). The gene RhCE encodes antigens named C, c, E and e. Note that 'c' and 'e' are real antigens and not just the absence of an antigen, like 'd'. Alternate gene splicing of RhCE produces two proteins.

D antigen is the strongest immunogen. Rh positive individuals are DD or Dd, Rh negative individuals are dd. Approximately 85% of Caucasians are Rh positive and 15% are Rh negative.

Anti-D antibodies are only generated when an Rh negative individual is exposed to Rh positive red cells following transfusion or pregnancy. All anti-D antibodies are IgG. Approximately 70% of Rh negative individuals produce anti-D antibodies after receiving Rh positive blood and they could develop transfusion reactions when re-transfused with Rh positive blood.

RhD haemolytic disease of the newborn

If blood from an Rh positive fetus enters the circulation of an Rh negative mother, sensitization can occur. Small amounts of fetal blood are transferred during the third trimester and at birth. Mothers develop anti-D IgG antibodies, which cross the placenta into the fetal circulation during the course of the second pregnancy. If the second fetus is Rh positive, the IgG antibodies induce immune haemolysis of fetal red cells, which can result in hydrops fetalis.

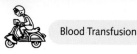
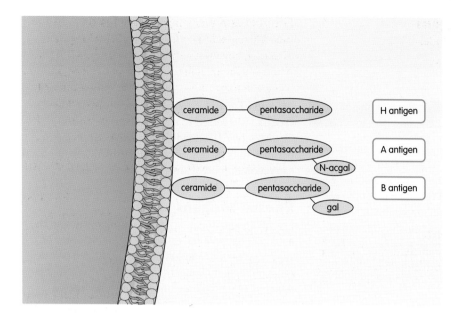

Fig. 8.1 ABO antigens (*N*-acgal, *N*-acetyl galactosamine; gal, galactose).

ABO blood groups		
Phenotype/Red cell antigens	**Genotype**	**Antibodies**
O	OO	Anti-A and Anti-B
A	AO or AA	Anti-B
B	BO or BB	Anti-A
AB	AB	None

Fig. 8.2 ABO blood groups.

Rhesus genotypes	
CDE genotype	**RhD**
cde/cde	Negative
CDe/cde	Positive
CDe/CDe	Positive
cDE/cde	Positive
CDe/cDE	Positive
cDE/cDE	Positive
Others	Most are positive

Fig. 8.3 Rhesus genotypes.

Prevention of RhD haemolytic disease of the newborn

Passive immunization is utilized to prevent maternal anti-D antibody production. The mother is given an intramuscular injection of anti-D IgG at 28 weeks and within 72 hours of the birth. The injected antibody coats Rh positive fetal red blood cells, which are removed by the reticuloendothelial system (RES) before the mother produces her own anti-D antibodies. The dose of anti-D IgG can be adjusted depending on the volume of fetal red blood cells in the maternal circulation, as estimated by the Kleihauer technique. Anti-D antibody is also used following abortion in Rh negative women and following transfusion of Rh positive blood into Rh negative individuals.

Red-cell antigens other than rhesus D, such as Kell and ABO incompatibility can also cause haemolytic disease of the newborn. ABO incompatibility leading to haemolytic disease of the newborn may occur during the first pregnancy; however, therapy should be given during every pregnancy to avoid problems.

Other red-cell antigens

Other red-cell antigens include:
- P
- Lewis
- I
- MN
- Kell
- Duffy
- Kidd.

Cross-matching and blood transfusion

Cross-matching blood

It is important to correctly identify the patient and to label samples accurately before blood transfusions to prevent potentially fatal transfusion reactions. Cross-matching has three stages:
1. Blood grouping (ABO and Rh) of the recipient
2. Screening for abnormal recipient antibodies
   - indirect antiglobulin test: the recipient's serum is tested against a standard pool of red cells to detect antibodies to blood group antigens other than those of the ABO and Rh systems
   - screening cells and cell panels.
3. Each unit of donor blood to be transfused is then tested against the patient's serum to identify atypical antibodies.

Emergency transfusions

Patients requiring emergency transfusions, e.g. for acute haemorrhage, should receive plasma-depleted red cells. Red cells are suspended in SAG-M (saline–adenine–glucose–mannitol—a nutrient solution). This contains little plasma and therefore reduces the risk of transfusing blood group antibodies or proteins.

Filtering and warming at transfusion

Blood-giving sets have filters with holes $170\mu m$ in diameter, however, very little is filtered out. Prior to current techniques in the processing of blood, filtering was needed to remove many unwanted components, including cell fragments. Blood is warmed when it is rapidly transfused to prevent vasoconstriction, which would reduce the rate of transfusion.

Dangers in the use of blood products
Transfusion reaction

Transfusion reactions occur when incompatible blood is transfused. A summary of the complications of blood transfusions is given in Fig. 8.4.

Haemolytic transfusion reactions

The most severe transfusion reaction, acute haemolysis, is caused by the destruction of donor red blood cells by antibodies (IgG or IgM) present in the recipient's serum. Haemolysis caused by IgM occurs immediately, reactions caused by IgG are delayed:
- Extravascular haemolysis results from incompatibilities of blood groups that produce IgG antibodies, e.g. Rh, Kell, Duffy and Kidd. Antibody-coated red blood cells are then removed by the RES
- ABO incompatibility (usually due to a clerical error) causes intravascular haemolysis when IgM antibodies fix complement. Activation of complement generates C3a and C5a, which cause vasodilatation, increased vascular permeability and neutrophil chemotaxis.

Symptoms can occur within a few minutes or may take several hours to develop. They include:
- Pain
- Fever

Fig. 8.4 Complications of blood transfusions. CMV, cytomegalovirus; HIV, human immunodeficiency virus.

Complications of blood transfusions	
Early	**Late**
Haemolytic reactions (immediate/delayed)	Transfusion transmitted infection
Allergic reactions to white cells, platelets or proteins (e.g. urticaria, anaphylaxis)	• Viral (e.g. CMV, HIV, hepatitis)
Febrile reactions	• Bacterial (e.g. *Salmonella*)
Transfusion related acute lung injury	• Parasites (e.g. malaria, *Toxoplasma*)
Circulatory overload	Iron overload
Air embolism	Alloimmunization (might cause rhesus
Thrombophlebitis	haemolytic disease in the future)
Hyperkalaemia	Graft-versus-host disease
Clotting abnormalities	

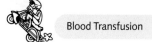

- Flushing
- Urticaria
- Headache
- Shortness of breath
- Rigors
- Diarrhoea and vomiting.

Release of vasoactive substances causes profound hypotension and shock, and renal tubular necrosis can cause acute renal failure. Release of tissue thromboplastin from lysed red cells can lead to disseminated intravascular coagulation (DIC). Death occurs in 15% of cases of ABO incompatibility and usually results from severe DIC or renal failure.

Blood products and infection risk

Infections have been transmitted in blood products. To minimize infection risk, donor blood is screened for several infective agents including syphilis, hepatitis B and C, and HIV.

Detection techniques are not foolproof. For example, HIV is detected by the presence of antibodies in donor blood. HIV has been transmitted in blood products from donors who had not seroconverted at the time of donation. Blood is taken aseptically and is then leucodepleted to reduce the risk of transmission.

There is concern about the transmission of variant Creutzfeldt–Jakob disease (vCJD). There is no reliable screening test or inactivation technique for vCJD, however, so far there have not been any reported cases of transmission in blood products.

Iron overload

The levels of iron in the body are usually controlled by the regulation of absorption. There are no physiological mechanisms to eliminate iron from the body. When people receive multiple blood transfusions, the excess iron is deposited in and causes damage to the heart, liver and endocrine organs. Iron-chelating agents, such as desferrioxamine and desferiprone facilitate iron excretion.

Other blood products
Platelets

Platelets are stored at room temperature (on an oscillating tray to prevent clumping) and have a half-life of 4–5 days. They can be obtained from a pool of 6–10 blood donors or from a single donor via apheresis. Indications for platelet transfusion include:

- Patients who are bleeding and who have a platelet count $<50 \times 10^9/L$
- Following massive transfusion resulting in dilutional thrombocytopenia
- Patients with platelet dysfunction who are bleeding
- Prophylactically in patients with thrombocytopenia who are undergoing surgery or who have bone marrow failure.

Fresh-frozen plasma

Fresh-frozen plasma (FFP) contains albumin, immunoglobulins and all the clotting factors. Indications for FFP transfusion include:

- Multiple clotting factor deficiencies, e.g. severe liver disease, warfarin overdose, massive transfusion (more than 10 units within 24 hours), thrombotic thrombocytopenic purpura
- Specific coagulation factor replacement
- Plasma loss (albumin solution is used in many cases, e.g. burns).

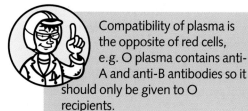

Compatibility of plasma is the opposite of red cells, e.g. O plasma contains anti-A and anti-B antibodies so it should only be given to O recipients.

Cryoprecipitate

Cryoprecipitate is the insoluble precipitate formed when FFP is thawed at 4°C. It contains factors VIII, vWF, factor XIII and fibrinogen, and is given to control bleeding associated with defects thereof. Cryoprecipitate can also be of use in chronic renal failure, advanced liver failure, disseminated intravascular failure and following massive blood transfusion.

Clotting factor concentrates

Specific clotting factor concentrates can be given to patients with clotting factor deficiencies (see Chapter 6).

White cells

Granulocyte concentrates can be given to infected neutropenic patients not responding to antibiotic therapy, but this is rare because of the risk of cytomegalovirus (CMV) transmission.

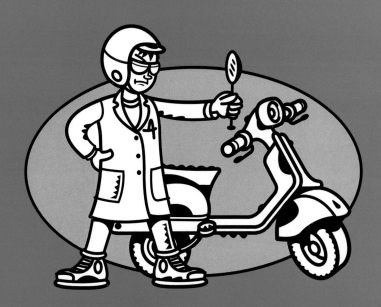

SELF-ASSESSMENT

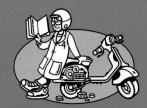

Indicate whether each answer is true or false.

1. Which of the following characteristics of tumour cells can activate an immune response:

(a) Viral antigens.
(b) Embryonic antigens.
(c) Glycosylated variants of normal self-proteins.
(d) Absence of MHC class I molecules.
(e) High concentrations of normal self-proteins.

2. Regarding the immune system:

(a) An antigen is a molecule that can be recognised by the adaptive immune system.
(b) Antibody isotypes are antibodies that bind to other antibodies.
(c) Haptens are not immunogenic by themselves.
(d) Lymph nodes are primary lymphoid organs.
(e) The innate immune system exhibits immunological memory.

3. In comparison to monocytes, macrophages:

(a) Are smaller.
(b) Live longer.
(c) Have greater phagocytic ability.
(d) Are more likely to be found in the circulation.
(e) Produce more lytic enzymes.

4. Macrophages can be activated by:

(a) Interferon-γ.
(b) Complement.
(c) Coagulation products.
(d) Interleukin-2.
(e) Fas ligand.

5. In comparison to macrophages, neutrophils:

(a) Are longer lived.
(b) Can control mycobacteria.
(c) Communicate with T cells.
(d) Can present exogenous antigen.
(e) Move and phagocytose more quickly.

6. Which of the following are products of oxygen-dependent pathways:

(a) Superoxide radicals.
(b) Hypochlorus acid.
(c) Lysozyme.
(d) Hydrogen peroxide.
(e) Cationic proteins.

7. Concerning natural killer cells:

(a) They are activated by specific, individual antigens.
(b) They can detect classical and non-classical MHC class I molecules.
(c) They are involved in antibody-dependent cell-mediated cytotoxicity.
(d) Because they are lymphoid cells, they exhibit immunological memory.
(e) They cause cellular necrosis.

8. Concerning the complement system:

(a) The classical pathway is activated by MHC molecules.
(b) It can be activated by bacterial carbohydrates.
(c) It can activate spontaneously.
(d) It causes ion-permeable pores to form in target cells.
(e) It is involved in the recruitment of inflammatory cells.

9. Which of the following inhibitors of complement are linked with the correct actions:

(a) Factor H inactivates C5 convertase.
(b) Decay accelerating factor speeds up the decay of the membrane attack complex.
(c) Factor I cleaves C3b and C4b.
(d) CD59 prevents the membrane attack complex from forming.
(e) C1 inhibitor inhibits C1.

10. Which of the following are members of the immunoglobulin gene superfamily:

(a) T cell receptor.
(b) CD3-ζ.
(c) Human leucocyte antigen molecules.
(d) ICAM-1.
(e) Polyimmunoglobulin receptor.

11. Concerning primary and secondary lymphoid tissue:

(a) The thymus is a secondary lymphoid organ.
(b) Lymph node germinal follicles contain mainly T cells.
(c) B-cell hypermutation occurs in the bone marrow.
(d) Lymph nodes sample antigen from the blood.
(e) Peyer's patches are part of the mucosal-associated lymphoid tissue.

12. Concerning generation of antigen receptor diversity:

(a) Both the light and heavy immunoglobulin chain variable regions are encoded by V, D and J gene segments.
(b) Diversity can only be generated before encountering antigen.
(c) Somatic hypermutation occurs in both B and T cells.
(d) Antibodies produced late in an immune response have increased affinity for antigen.
(e) Each person's T cell receptor repertoire will be the same.

13. IgA:

(a) Is important in mucosal immunity.
(b) Is found in breast milk.
(c) Is the most abundant immunoglobulin in the blood.
(d) Crosses the placenta.
(e) Is normally a dimer.

14. The major histocompatibility complex (MHC):

(a) Encodes human leucocyte antigen (HLA) molecules.
(b) Is located on chromosome 16 in humans.
(c) Encodes some complement components.
(d) Contains the gene for TNF.
(e) Encodes β_2-microglobulin.

15. Concerning the acute phase response:

(a) There is a change in the concentration of a number of plasma proteins.
(b) Leucocytosis and thrombocytopenia develop.
(c) Levels of caeruloplasmin and α_1-glycoprotein undergo a 100–1000-fold increase.
(d) Levels of C-reactive protein and serum amyloid A rise within hours of tissue injury.
(e) There is a decrease in plasma viscosity.

16. Concerning class I MHC molecules:

(a) A class I molecule is made up of α- and β-chains.
(b) CD8$^+$ T cells are class I MHC-restricted.
(c) Class I molecules are present only on antigen-presenting cells.
(d) Class I molecules present endogenous antigen.
(e) A class I molecule can bind longer peptides than a class II molecule because the peptide-binding cleft is more open.

17. Concerning recognition molecules of the immune system:

(a) Immunoglobulin molecules consist of two heavy chains and two light chains.
(b) The variable regions of the heavy and light chains are identical.
(c) The framework regions of immunoglobulins comprise the antigen-binding site.
(d) TCR signals are transduced by Igα/Igβ.
(e) Approximately 95% of T cells express $\gamma\delta$ receptors.

18. The following are components of the innate immune system:

(a) Interferons α and β.
(b) T cells.
(c) Complement.
(d) Antibody.
(e) Acute phase proteins.

19. di George syndrome is characterized by:

(a) Malformation of the third and fourth pharyngeal pouches.
(b) Thymic hyperplasia.
(c) Hyperparathyroidism.
(d) Cardiac defects.
(e) Recurrent infections.

20. Regarding the complement system:

(a) Complement components are proteins or glycoproteins.
(b) Complement can only be activated by the alternative and classical pathways.
(c) The alternative pathway is usually activated by IgM and IgG.
(d) Complement components C5, C6, C7, C8 and C9 comprise the membrane attack complex.
(e) The conversion of C3 to C3b by C3 convertase is the major amplification process in the complement cascade.

21. Concerning lymph nodes:

(a) Antigen enters lymph nodes from the blood.
(b) Lymph filters from the cortex to the medulla.
(c) They contain B cells, T cells and antigen-presenting cells.
(d) Lymphocytes can enter the node directly from the blood.
(e) They act to pump lymph around the body.

22. The following are examples of mucosal-associated lymphoid tissue (MALT):

(a) Tonsils.
(b) Appendix.
(c) Thymus.
(d) Peyer's patches.
(e) Inguinal lymph nodes.

23. The thymus:

(a) Is a bilobed gland.
(b) Is usually located in the neck.
(c) Exhibits a high rate of cell death.
(d) Contains stromal cells that support developing neutrophils.
(e) Produces hormones that control T cell maturation.

24. T helper cells:

(a) Express CD4.
(b) Are required for antibody production against protein antigens.
(c) Produce a wide variety of cytokines, which stimulate the innate and adaptive immune systems.
(d) Do not express T cell receptors.
(e) Determine the type of adaptive immune response mounted.

25. Concerning acute inflammation:

(a) Acute inflammation is characterized by infiltration of neutrophils and vascular changes.
(b) TNF-α is an important mediator.
(c) The complement system does not play a role.
(d) The coagulation and fibrinolytic systems are activated.
(e) ICAM-1 and ICAM-2 are downregulated.

26. The actions of cytokines in acute inflammation include:

(a) Induction of adhesion molecules.
(b) Induction of cell membrane phospholipid and prostaglandin metabolism.
(c) Chemotaxis of neutrophils.
(d) Stimulate fibroblast proliferation.
(e) Mediate the acute phase response.

27. Which of the following are arachidonic acid metabolites:

(a) Platelet-activating factor.
(b) Leukotriene B$_4$.
(c) Thromboxane A$_2$.
(d) Perforin.
(e) Prostacyclin.

28. Concerning leucocyte margination and extravasation in acute inflammation:

(a) Neutrophils are important in the early part of the response.
(b) Selectin molecules expressed constitutively on endothelial cells bind to selectin molecules on leucocytes.
(c) The interaction between leucocytes and endothelium is strengthened by integrin molecules.
(d) Integrin molecules are important for leucocyte homing.
(e) The endothelial cells form pores large enough for spherical leucocytes to pass through.

29. Concerning chronic inflammation:

(a) Neutrophils form the majority of cells present.
(b) The macrophage plays a central role.
(c) Granuloma formation is a characteristic feature.
(d) TNF-α is crucial in granuloma maintenance.
(e) Lymphocytes are not usually present.

30. The following are potential consequences of chronic inflammation:

(a) Tissue injury.
(b) The tissue returns to normal.
(c) Weight loss and fever.
(d) Adaptive immune system activation.
(e) Fibrosis.

31. Which of the following are important for the immune response to viruses:

(a) Lysozyme.
(b) Antibody.
(c) Interferons.
(d) Eosinophils.
(e) Cytotoxic T cells.

32. Viruses evade the normal immune response by:

(a) Undergoing mutation between epidemics.
(b) Reducing MHC class I expression.
(c) Mutating within the host.
(d) Releasing exotoxins.
(e) Becoming latent.

33. Protozoal infection is often chronic because:

(a) They have marked antigenic variation.
(b) They are immunosuppressive.
(c) They have complex lifecycles.
(d) Infection is intracellular.
(e) They can escape into the cytoplasm following phagocytosis.

34. Regarding hypersensitivity reactions:

(a) Type I hypersensitivity reactions are mediated by IgG.
(b) Type III hypersensitivity involves the formation of immune complexes.
(c) Mast cells play a key role in immediate hypersensitivity.
(d) Delayed-type hypersensitivity mechanisms play a key role in haemolytic disease of the newborn due to rhesus incompatibility.
(e) The Arthus reaction is a localized type III reaction.

35. The following are examples of hypersensitivity reactions:

(a) A positive skin-prick test.
(b) A positive Mantoux or Heaf test.
(c) Hay fever.
(d) Graves' disease.
(e) Osteoarthritis.

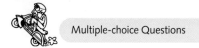

36. **Concerning anti-inflammatory drugs:**

(a) Paracetamol is an excellent anti-inflammatory.
(b) Steroids can only be given intravenously.
(c) NSAIDs act by inhibiting phospholipase A_2.
(d) Anti-TNF-α is anti-inflammatory.
(e) NSAIDs may be nephrotoxic and cause bronchospasm.

37. **Concerning allergies:**

(a) They are always type I hypersensitivity reactions.
(b) Asthma is characterized by reversible airway obstruction.
(c) Pollen and dust-mite faeces are common allergens.
(d) Atopy refers to a predisposition to allergic conditions.
(e) Anaphylaxis is associated with hypertension.

38. **Concerning treatment of allergies:**

(a) Controlled exposure to low doses of antigen can be helpful.
(b) Antihistamines cure many allergic conditions.
(c) Steroids are useful.
(d) Adrenaline is commonly needed in the treatment of severe anaphlyaxis.
(e) Prophylactic treatment often reduces the occurrence of symptoms.

39. **Self-tolerance can be due to:**

(a) Early clonal deletion.
(b) Clonal anergy.
(c) Molecular mimicry.
(d) Fas ligand expression.
(e) Regulatory T cells.

40. **Concerning systemic lupus erythematous (SLE):**

(a) SLE is an organ-specific autoimmune disease.
(b) SLE is more common in men than women.
(c) SLE is characterized by antinuclear autoantibodies.
(d) The presence of HLA-DR5 and HLA-DR6 haplotypes confers an increased risk of developing SLE.
(e) An erythematous rash is common.

41. **Concerning rheumatoid arthritis (RA):**

(a) RA is characterized by inflammation of the synovium and destruction of the articular cartilage.
(b) Inflammation is limited to joints.
(c) TNF is a key cytokine in pathogenesis.
(d) RA is more common in women than in men.
(e) Type II collagen is the major autoantigen.

42. **Rheumatoid factor:**

(a) Is found in all cases of rheumatoid arthritis.
(b) Is an autoantibody,
(c) Is directed against IgM.
(d) Can activate complement.
(e) Amplifies the inflammatory response.

43. **The following autoimmune diseases are organ specific:**

(a) Reiter's syndrome.
(b) Hashimoto's thyroiditis.
(c) Myasthenia gravis.
(d) Graves' disease.
(e) Polyarteritis nodosa.

44. **The following are examples of primary immunodeficiencies:**

(a) Chronic granulomatous disease.
(b) Transient hypogammaglobulinaemia of infancy.
(c) Splenectomy.
(d) AIDS.
(e) Wiskott–Aldrich syndrome.

45. **Antibody deficiency can present with:**

(a) Bronchiectasis.
(b) Diarrhoea.
(c) Rheumatoid arthritis.
(d) Hyperviscosity.
(e) Mycoplasma joint infections.

46. **Features of HIV include:**

(a) Polyclonal B cell activation.
(b) Defective T cell function.
(c) Low rate of viral replication during asymptomatic phase.
(d) Antibodies directed against gp120 and gp41.
(e) Persistent generalized lymphadenopathy.

47. **During HIV infection, which of the following infections are common:**

(a) CMV retinitis.
(b) *Pneumocystis carinii*.
(c) Oesophageal candidiasis.
(d) *Mycobacterium avium intracellulare* (MAC).
(e) Toxoplasmosis.

48. **Concerning the routine immunization schedule in the UK:**

(a) MMR is given at 2, 3 and 4 months.
(b) BCG is given neonatally or at 10–14 years.
(c) Influenza vaccine is given to people over 65 years of age.
(d) Meningococcal vaccine is given before the child goes to school.
(e) Tetanus vaccine require boosters.

49. **Live vaccines are used to prevent:**

(a) Polio.
(b) Tetanus.
(c) Tuberculosis.
(d) Rubella.
(e) Hepatitis B.

50. Concerning mechanisms of transplant rejection:

(a) Hyperacute rejection only occurs once the recipient has synthesized antibody to the graft.
(b) Acute cellular rejection is primarily mediated by natural killer cells.
(c) Acute rejection is due to anti-donor antibodies.
(d) Chronic rejection may be due to several mechanisms.
(e) Complement is implicated in hyperacute rejection.

51. The risk of transplant rejection can be reduced by:

(a) Using a graft from a monozygous twin.
(b) Using steroids.
(c) Using monoclonal antibodies.
(d) Prompt cooling of transplanted organs.
(e) Using unmatched grafts.

52. Bone marrow:

(a) Is the main site of haemopoiesis in adults.
(b) Is found throughout the skeleton of newborns.
(c) Contains a large amount of fat.
(d) Contains macrophages important for the transfer of iron to developing erythrocytes.
(e) Forms T lymphocyte precursors.

53. Regarding the spleen:

(a) The spleen is normally anterior to the stomach.
(b) The red pulp removes old or defective erythrocytes from the circulation.
(c) There are usually more primary than secondary B cell follicles.
(d) Develops from the primitive gut.
(e) Primary cancers are rare.

54. Haematopoietic stem cells:

(a) Are found only in the bone marrow.
(b) Are able to produce plasma cells.
(c) Can self replicate.
(d) Become lineage-committed precursor cells.
(e) Need growth factors to differentiate.

55. Concerning disorders of the spleen:

(a) Congestive splenomegaly is caused by persistent venous congestion.
(b) Splenomegaly in the UK is usually due to parasitic infection.
(c) Splenic infarction occurs in myeloproliferative disorders.
(d) Epstein–Barr virus infection is linked to splenic rupture.
(e) The spleen may be affected by haematological neoplasms.

56. Splenectomy is indicated in:

(a) Splenic rupture.
(b) Splenic tumours.
(c) Idiopathic thrombocytopenic purpura.
(d) Autoimunne haemolytic anaemia.
(e) Splenic cysts.

57. Hereditary spherocytosis is characterized by:

(a) An autosomal dominant pattern of inheritance.
(b) Intravascular haemolysis.
(c) The presence of spherocytes on the peripheral blood film smear.
(d) Increased osmotic fragility of red cells.
(e) Decreased autohaemolysis of red cells.

58. Features of β-thalassaemia major include:

(a) A microcytic, hypochromic anaemia.
(b) High serum iron.
(c) Increased red-cell lifespan.
(d) Homozygosity for defective genes causing reduced β-chain production.
(e) HbA on electrophoresis.

59. Erythrocytes:

(a) Have a bilobed nucleus.
(b) Are derived from the CFU-GEMM precursor.
(c) Transport CO_2.
(d) Have an average life span of 50 days.
(e) Are usually spherical.

60. Concerning iron metabolism:

(a) Iron is absorbed in the stomach.
(b) Excess iron is readily excreted.
(c) Iron is transported in the blood bound to apoferritin.
(d) Primary haemochromatosis is caused by excessive intestinal absorption.
(e) Total body stores of iron are 4 kg.

61. Concerning haemoglobin:

(a) Adult haemoglobin is composed of four identical polypeptide subunits.
(b) Oxygen is transported bound to haem.
(c) The Bohr effect (a shift of the oxygen dissociation curve) is due to increased H^+.
(d) Oxygen binding follows a sigmoidal curve.
(e) 2,3-diphosphoglycerate levels rise in hypoxia to allow increased oxygen uptake by haemoglobin.

62. Vitamin B$_{12}$:

(a) Is absorbed in the proximal jejunum.
(b) Contains cobalt.
(c) Absorption is reduced following total gastrectomy.
(d) Requires extrinsic factor for absorption.
(e) Is synthesized by the skin.

63. Regarding folic acid:

(a) It is found in vegetables.
(b) It is absorbed in the colon.
(c) 50mg per day is the normal daily requirement.
(d) Deficiency may occur in coeliac disease.
(e) The requirement decreases during pregnancy.

64. A normochromic normocytic anaemia is commonly associated with:

(a) Iron deficiency.
(b) Tuberculosis.
(c) Rheumatoid arthritis.
(d) Vitamin B_{12} deficiency.
(e) Thalassaemia.

65. Which of the following are features of iron-deficiency anaemia?

(a) Glossitis.
(b) Koilonychia.
(c) Macrocytic, hypochromic anaemia.
(d) Reduced serum ferritin.
(e) Reduced serum transferrin.

66. Causes of absolute polycythaemia include:

(a) Polycythaemia rubra vera.
(b) Dehydration.
(c) Renal carcinoma.
(d) Cyanotic heart disease.
(e) Diuretic therapy.

67. Which of the following are red-cell precursors:

(a) Pronormoblast.
(b) Normoblast.
(c) Stomatocyte.
(d) Reticulocyte.
(e) Echinocyte.

68. Which of the following are features of haemolytic anaemias:

(a) Pigment gallstones.
(b) Raised serum haptoglobin.
(c) Haemosiderinuria.
(d) Haemoglobinaemia.
(e) Reticulocytosis.

69. Which of the following can precipitate haemolysis in glucose-6-phosphate dehydrogenase deficiency?

(a) Infection.
(b) Alkalosis.
(c) Primaquine.
(d) Fava beans.
(e) Normal saline.

70. Management of sickle-cell anaemia can include:

(a) Vaccinations.
(b) Folic acid.
(c) Antibiotics.
(d) Blood transfusions.
(e) Fluids.

71. Fetal haemoglobin:

(a) Has a sigmoidal oxygen dissociation curve.
(b) Has a lower affinity for oxygen than adult haemoglobin.
(c) May be raised in β-thalassaemia syndromes.
(d) Is produced by the fetal liver.
(e) Is composed of two α and two β chains.

72. Erythropoietin:

(a) Prevents apoptosis of developing erythrocyte precursors.
(b) Is produced in the bone marrow.
(c) Is raised in chronic hypoxia.
(d) May be used iatrogenically.
(e) Is needed for white cell maturation.

73. Aplastic anaemia can be:

(a) Iatrogenic.
(b) Part of a congenital syndrome.
(c) Associated with acute infection.
(d) Associated with increased bone marrow cellularity.
(e) Treated with testosterone.

74. In haemolytic anaemia:

(a) Red-cell fragmentation can be associated with prosthetic heart valves.
(b) Acute renal failure can occur.
(c) Urinary bilirubin is increased.
(d) Urinary urobilinogen is increased.
(e) A microcytosis is common.

75. Polymorphonuclear leucocytes:

(a) Have a large round nucleus.
(b) Primarily respond to parasitic infections.
(c) Are granulocytes.
(d) Are phagocytic.
(e) Are a major constituent of pus.

76. Myelodysplastic syndromes:

(a) Are acquired neoplastic disorders of the bone marrow.
(b) Are due to defects in fully differentiated cells.
(c) May progress to acute myeloid leukaemia.
(d) Are commonest in children.
(e) Have a worse prognosis when blasts account for more than 5% of the bone marrow.

77. Leucostatic symptoms:

(a) Occur in leukaemia.
(b) Are caused by fat embolism.
(c) Include retinal haemorrhage.
(d) Include reduced level of consciousness.
(e) Resolve if the white-cell count increases.

78. Which of the following are consistent with a diagnosis of non-Hodgkin's lymphoma:

(a) Painless lymphadenopathy.
(b) Reed–Sternberg cells in the lesion.
(c) Fever, night sweats and weight loss.
(d) Fanconi's syndrome.
(e) HIV infection.

79. Which of the following are myeloproliferative conditions:

(a) Polycythaemia rubra vera.
(b) Sideroblastic anaemia.
(c) Myelofibrosis.
(d) Primary thrombocythaemia.
(e) Acute lymphoblastic leukaemia.

80. A macrophage:

(a) Is a differentiated monocyte.
(b) Is capable of phagocytosis.
(c) May play an important role in the adaptive immune response.
(d) Can be infected by HIV.
(e) Is central to the allergic response.

81. Chronic lymphocytic leukaemia:

(a) Is the most common leukaemia.
(b) Is rapidly progressive.
(c) Is usually B cell in origin.
(d) Is commonly associated with autoimmune haemolytic anaemia.
(e) Converts to acute leukaemia within 5 years.

82. Regarding acute lymphoblastic leukaemia:

(a) It is the most common leukaemia in children.
(b) Presentation after 10 years of age is associated with a poorer prognosis.
(c) Remission rates are low.
(d) It is commonly T cell in origin.
(e) It may be caused by radiation exposure.

83. Acute myeloblastic leukaemia:

(a) Is caused by an accumulation of differentiated myeloid cells in the bone marrow.
(b) Is associated with Down syndrome.
(c) Is characterized by isochromosome 12p.
(d) Has a better prognosis in older patients.
(e) May present with bleeding.

84. Regarding chronic myeloid leukaemia:

(a) It is often identified in chronic phase.
(b) Less than 10% of patients develop to an accelerated phase within 10 years of diagnosis.
(c) The Philadelphia chromosome is a disease marker.
(d) Treatment may be with Glivec.
(e) Bone marrow transplant is potentially curative.

85. Which of the following are features of multiple myeloma:

(a) Bence-Jones protein in the plasma.
(b) Presentation with paraplegia.
(c) Repeated infections.
(d) Bone destruction.
(e) >10% plasma cells in the marrow.

86. Which of the following may cause a neutropenia:

(a) Aplastic anaemia.
(b) Leukaemia.
(c) Kostmann's syndrome.
(d) Chemotherapy.
(e) Antimalarial drugs.

87. Platelets:

(a) Are derived from the nucleus of megakaryocytes.
(b) Are transported in the blood by von Willebrand's factor.
(c) Are involved in primary haemostasis.
(d) Can bind directly to collagen.
(e) Are inhibited by thromboxane A_2.

88. Bleeding can occur as a consequence of:

(a) Drug therapy.
(b) Chemotherapy and radiotherapy.
(c) X-linked diseases.
(d) Splenomegaly.
(e) Defective platelet adhesion.

89. Concerning vitamin-K-dependent clotting factors:

(a) Prothrombin is a vitamin-K-dependent clotting factor.
(b) Factor IX is vitamin K dependent.
(c) Vitamin K is required for post-translational acetylation.
(d) Vitamin K deficiency can be caused by fat malabsorption.
(e) Haemophilia A can be caused by vitamin K deficiency.

90. Which of the following will cause the prothrombin time to be increased:

(a) Disseminated intravascular coagulation.
(b) von Willebrand's disease.
(c) Vitamin K deficiency.
(d) Haemophilia A.
(e) Haemophilia B.

91. Which of the following are associated with an increased risk of clotting:

(a) Factor V Leiden.
(b) Disseminated cancer.
(c) Oestrogen therapy.
(d) Protein C deficiency.
(e) Prolonged immobilization.

92. Idiopathic thrombocytopenic purpura:

(a) Is characterized by IgA-positive petechiae.
(b) Is associated with anti-platelet antibodies in the plasma.
(c) Is associated with HIV disease.
(d) May be treated with high-dose glucocorticoids.
(e) May be treated with fresh-frozen plasma only.

93. Heparin:

(a) Is routinely given orally.
(b) Is routinely monitored using the international normalized ratio.
(c) Is a glycosaminoglycan.
(d) Has a different activity at different molecular weights.
(e) Is structurally related to warfarin.

94. Which of the following limit thrombus formation:

(a) Proteins C and S.
(b) Plasminogen activator inhibitor.
(c) Thrombocytopenia.
(d) Streptokinase.
(e) Christmas factor.

95. Regarding haemophilia A:

(a) Inheritance is autosomal dominant.
(b) Prevalence depends on social class.
(c) It may be treated prophylactically with factor VII.
(d) It is associated with pathological arthrodesis.
(e) It may be mimicked by von Willebrand's disease.

96. Which of the following test results are in the normal range for peripheral venous blood in a healthy 25-year-old man:

(a) Haemoglobin: 14 g/dL.
(b) White-cell count: 8×10^9/L.
(c) pO_2: 40 mmHg.
(d) Reticulocyte count: 5% of peripheral red blood cells.
(e) Platelets: 100×10^9/L.

97. Which of the following are detected on peripheral blood smears:

(a) Howell–Jolly bodies.
(b) Auer rods.
(c) Philadelphia chromosome.
(d) Reticulocytosis.
(e) Bence-Jones protein.

98. Regarding the ABO antigen system:

(a) People who are blood group O must have two parents who are both blood group O.
(b) People who are blood group A will produce anti-B antibodies.
(c) In group O, the T antigen is left unchanged.
(d) Group AB people will usually produce a haemolytic reaction to group O blood.
(e) Anti-A and anti-B antibodies are usually IgG.

99. Haemolytic disease of the newborn:

(a) Is commonly due to rhesus D incompatibility.
(b) Usually occurs in the first child.
(c) Will not occur if the mother is rhesus D positive.
(d) Can be prevented by passive immunization.
(e) Is due to IgM antibodies.

100. Regarding acute haemolytic transfusion reactions:

(a) They are caused by the destruction of donor red blood cells by antibodies present in the recipient's serum.
(b) They may lead to complement activation.
(c) They develop a few days after transfusion.
(d) Hypertension, flushing, urticaria, diarrhoea and vomiting ensue.
(e) They may cause disseminated intravascular coagulation.

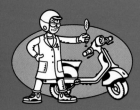

Short-answer Questions (SAQs)

1. What are the differences between Th1 and Th2 cells?

_____

2. Explain what the term 'positive and negative selection of T cells' means and state where these processes take place.

_____

3. List the clinical features of haemolytic anaemias and explain how they arise.

_____

4. Draw the structure of an immunoglobulin molecule and list the functions of immunoglobulins.

_____

5. Write short notes on pernicious anaemia.

_____

6. What is haemolytic disease of the newborn and how can it be prevented?

_____

7. Define the following terms: innate and adaptive immunity; antigen; immunogen; hapten; epitope.

_____

8. What are the differences between active and passive immunization? Outline the advantages and disadvantages of each.

_____

9. Write short notes on the role of vitamin K in coagulation.

_____

10. Draw and label a diagram of a platelet.

_____

11. A 24-year-old intravenous drug abuser presents to casualty with weight loss, fever and 2 months of unproductive cough. A chest radiograph reveals bilateral hilar lymphadenopathy. A full blood count showed a haemoglobin of 8 g/dL with a normal neutrophil count and a total lymphocyte count of 0.1.
    (i)   What is the most likely diagnosis?
    (ii) How else may a patient with this condition have presented?
    (iii) What medications are available to treat his underlying condition?

12. A 65-year-old man presents with diffuse symmetrical lymphadenopathy and splenomegaly. He complains only of tiredness. A full blood count reveals a haemoglobin of 9 g/dL (normochromic, normocytic), his total leucocyte count is 125×10^9/L, composed mostly of lymphocytes.
    (i)   What is the most likely diagnosis?
    (ii) How would you establish this diagnosis?
    (iii) How would you treat him, and what is his prognosis?

13. A 57-year-old man with lumbar back pain of 2 weeks duration is brought into casualty paraplegic after a minor fall. X-ray showed osteolytic lesions with vertebral collapse, and protein electrophoresis showed a paraprotein in his serum.
    (i)   What is the most likely diagnosis?
    (ii) What other clinical features might you expect this patient to exhibit?

14. A 15-year-old male presents with chronic sputum production and is found to have thickened bronchial walls on chest CT. The appearances are consistent with bronchiectasis. He also complains of recurrent gastrointestinal infections. His father died from bronchiectasis at the age of 35.
    (i)   What is the likely diagnosis?
    (ii) What treatment would you offer him?

15. You are involved in the care of a 20-year-old man who was involved in a motorbike accident and rushed to casualty by ambulance. Amongst his injuries he had fractured his 10th rib on the left hand side. The fractured bone had ruptured his spleen and it was necessary to perform an emergency splenectomy. What advice would you give him about his prognosis?

16. A 63-year-old Caucasian woman presents with a severe pyrexia of unknown origin. She has irregular peaks of fever and profound malaise. Investigations revealed a CRP of 300mg/L (normal 10mg/L), haemoglobin 9g/dL (normochromic, normocytic), albumin 14g/L (35–50g/L) and polyclonal gammopathy. A chest CT taken 1 month previously revealed diffuse basal reticular shadowing, which, on repeat CT, progressed rapidly in parallel with the patient's requirement for oxygen. All microbiological tests on bronchio-alveolar lavage were negative and a transbronchial biopsy was negative. Bone marrow showed reactive changes only.
    (i) What test would you perform to establish the diagnosis?
    (ii) What possible diagnoses might this test reveal?

17. An 18-year-old haemophiliac who has been well maintained haematologically in the UK went to Nepal following his A-levels. During this time he fell over and required treatment with blood products exceeding those he had taken with him. He presents with fever, maculopapular rash, splenomegaly and mouth ulcers 8 weeks after returning to the UK. He is severely lymphopenic with normal polymorphonuclear count and haemogloblin.
    (i) What blood products may he have received?
    (ii) What prime diagnosis must be excluded?

18. A 20-year-old white Caucasian male who had dropped out of university, was sent by his mother to a health food farm where he received a diet of broad beans. Two days after arriving he developed jaundice but initially had normal coloured urine, which changed to red after 1 day.
    (i) What is the likely diagnosis?
    (ii) What would urine tests show?
    (iii) What would be the salient changes in blood tests?

19. A 40-year-old man presents with a right hemiplegia. On examination he has a ruddy complexion and no movement in his right arm and leg. He has no previous history of serious disease. He is afebrile, has no cardiac murmurs and is not hypertensive.
    (i) What is the first urgent test you require and why?
    (ii) Polycythaemia rubra vera is considered likely. What other investigations should you carry out?
    (iii) If a diagnosis of polycythaemia rubra vera was confirmed, how would you manage this patient?

20. A 15-year-old bee-keeper's daughter presents to casualty 15 minutes after being stung by a bee. She has severely obstructed breathing caused by laryngeal oedema and is becoming cyanosed.
    (i) What is the most likely diagnosis?
    (ii) How would you treat her?

Essay Questions

1. Describe the different mechanisms that operate to generate diversity of the B- and T-cell antigen receptors.

2. Compare and contrast the structure and function of a macrophage and a neutrophil.

3. Write an essay on the red cell cytoskeleton. What happens if it is defective?

4. Relate the structure of the immunoglobulin molecule to its functions.

5. Discuss the treatment of rheumatoid arthritis, explaining how the knowledge of pathophysiology has been utilized.

6. Write an essay on sickle-cell anaemia, with special reference to the pathogenesis, clinical features and laboratory findings.

7. Compare and contrast the process of acute and chronic inflammation.

8. Compare and contrast the innate and adaptive immune systems.

9. Describe the process by which blood is cross-matched prior to transfusion. What happens if an O-negative patient receives blood from an AB-positive patient?

10. Describe the mechanisms that usually protect an individual from autoimmunity and discuss how they can breakdown.

11. How is coagulation regulated?

12. Describe the mechanisms that pathogens use to avoid the immune response.

13. Describe the process of natural killer (NK) cell activation, and explain how NK cells cause cytotoxicity.

14. Describe the process of haemopoiesis and its regulation.

15. Compare and contrast Hodgkin's and non-Hodgkin's lymphomas.

16. Write an essay on hypersensitivity, including the immunological mechanisms and examples.

17. Discuss the causes and management of aplastic anaemia.

18. Compare and contrast haemophilia A, haemophilia B and von Willebrand's disease.

19. Discuss the factors involved in controlling white cells leaving the circulation.

20. Describe the clinical presentation of leukaemia.

MCQ Answers

1.
(a) T—Tumours induced by viral infection can express viral antigens.
(b) T—Carcino-embryonic antigen is seen in colonic cancer; α-fetoprotein in liver cancers.
(c) T—Normal cell proteins can become abnormally glycosylated in tumours.
(d) T—Absence of MHC class I can stimulate NK cells.
(e) F—Completely normal proteins cannot stimulate the immune system.

2.
(a) T—Antigens are recognized by the adaptive immune system.
(b) F—Isotypes are different classes of antibody.
(c) T—Haptens require large carrier molecules to elicit an immune response.
(d) F—Lymph nodes are secondary lymphoid organs.
(e) F—The innate immune system does not exhibit memory.

3.
(a) F—Macrophages are larger than monocytes.
(b) T—Macrophages can survive for many years within the tissues.
(c) T—Macrophages are primarily phagocytic.
(d) F—Macrophages form from monocytes when they enter tissues.
(e) T—Lytic enzymes are produced to improve destruction of phagocytosed material.

4.
(a) T—Cytokines, including IFN-γ, activate macrophages.
(b) T—Complement acts as an opsonin for phagocytes.
(c) T—Coagulation products activate macrophages.
(d) F—IL-2 is a T-cell growth factor.
(e) F—Fas ligand will cause cells expressing Fas to undergo apoptosis.

5.
(a) F—Macrophages are longer lived, neutrophils die soon after dealing with pathogens.
(b) F—Macrophages are required to control mycobacteria.
(c) F—Macrophages, but not neutrophils, stimulate T cells by secreting IL-12.
(d) F—Neutrophils do not process exogenous antigen or produce MHC class II to present antigen.
(e) T—Neutrophils move and phagocytose more quickly then macrophages.

6.
(a) T—Superoxide radicals are produced from molecular oxygen.
(b) T—Hypochlorus acid is produced when myeloperoxidase catalyses a reaction between hydrogen peroxide and chloride ions.
(c) F—Lysozyme is oxygen independent and acts to split peptidoglycan.
(d) T—Hydrogen peroxide is formed when superoxide radicals combine with hydrogen ions.
(e) F—Cationic proteins are oxygen independent and damage microbial membranes.

7.
(a) F—Natural killer cells do not recognize specific individual antigens, but characteristics of cells such as the level of MHC expression.
(b) T—KIRs detect classical MHC class I; CD94:NKG2 detects non-classical MHC class I.
(c) T—Natural killer cells can kill antibody-coated cells irrespective of the presence of MHC.
(d) F—Natural killer cells are part of the innate immune system and do not exhibit memory.
(e) F—Killing is via apoptosis.

8.
(a) F—The classical pathway is activated by antibody bound to antigen.
(b) T—The lectin pathway is activated when mannan-binding lectin binds to bacterial carbohydrates.
(c) T—The alternative pathway starts with spontaneous activation of C3.
(d) T—Complement killing is by formation of the membrane attack complex.
(e) T—Complement recruits inflammatory cells and kills or opsonizes pathogens.

9.
(a) F—Factor H prevents assembly of C3 convertase.
(b) F—Decay accelerating factor accelerates the decay of C3 convertase.
(c) T—Factor I and membrane cofactor protein cleave C3b and C4b.
(d) T—CD59 (protectin) prevents the membrane attack complex forming.
(e) T—C1 inhibitor inhibits C1.

10.
(a) T—The T cell receptor consists of four immunoglobulin domains.
(b) F—CD3-ε, γ and δ contain immunoglobulin domains but ζ does not.
(c) T—HLA molecules consist of four immunoglobulin domains.
(d) T—Certain adhesion molecules, including ICAM-1, are members of the immunoglobulin gene superfamily.
(e) T—The polyimmunoglobulin receptor is a member of the immunoglobulin gene superfamily.

11. (a) F—T cell maturation occurs in the thymus, therefore it is a primary lymphoid organ.
    (b) F—Lymph node germinal follicles are primarily composed of B cells.
    (c) F—Diversity in immunoglobulin molecules is generated in the bone marrow, but somatic hypermutation occurs within germinal centres.
    (d) F—Lymph nodes sample antigen from lymph (fluid drained from interstitial tissues).
    (e) T—Peyer's patches are organized mucosal-associated lymphoid organs.

12. (a) F—The light chain has only V and J segments.
    (b) F—Somatic hypermutation of immunoglobulin occurs after encountering antigen.
    (c) F—T cells do not undergo somatic hypermutation.
    (d) T—Antibody affinity increases during an immune response because of somatic hypermutation.
    (e) F—The T cell receptor repertoire depends on HLA molecules, which are polymorphic.

13. (a) T—IgA is secreted across mucosal surfaces.
    (b) T—IgA is also secreted in breast milk.
    (c) F—IgG is the most abundant immunoglobulin in blood.
    (d) F—IgG, not IgA, crosses the placenta.
    (e) T—IgA is usually dimeric.

14. (a) T—HLA molecules are human MHC molecules.
    (b) F—The HLA complex is found on chromosome 6.
    (c) T—The class III region of HLA encodes C4 and C2.
    (d) T—The TNF gene is encoded within the MHC.
    (e) F—β_2-microglobulin is not encoded on chromosome 6.

15. (a) T—The acute phase plasma proteins increase in concentration.
    (b) F—Thrombocytosis develops.
    (c) F—Levels of caeruloplasmin rise to about 150% of normal levels.
    (d) T—CRP and SAA rise rapidly.
    (e) F—Plasma viscosity and ESR are raised.

16. (a) F—Class I molecules are formed from α-chains and β_2-microglobulin.
    (b) T—CD8$^+$ T cells are class I MHC-restricted, targeting them to endogenous antigen presentation.
    (c) F—All nucleated cells express class I molecules.
    (d) T—Class I molecules present endogenous antigen.
    (e) F—Class I molecules present peptides 9 amino acids long, class II present peptides 12–15 peptides long.

17. (a) T—Each immunoglobulin molecule consists of two identical heavy chains and two identical light chains.
    (b) F—The variable regions of the heavy and light chains are derived from different genetic recombination events.
    (c) F—The variable regions comprise the antigen-binding site.
    (d) F—TCR signals through CD3.
    (e) F—Approximately 5% of T cells express $\alpha\beta$ receptors.

18. (a) T—Interferons α and β are produced by a wide number of cells to induce an antiviral state (γ-interferon is produced by T cells).
    (b) F—T cells are part of the adaptive immune response.
    (c) T—The complement system is a cascade of proteins involved in the innate immune system.
    (d) F—Antibodies are specific and therefore part of the adaptive response.
    (e) T—Acute phase proteins are innate molecules.

19. (a) T—Malformation of the third and fourth pharyngeal pouches can lead to failure of thymic development.
    (b) F—In di George syndrome the thymus is hypoplastic.
    (c) F—The parathyroid glands also fail to develop.
    (d) T—Cardiac defects occurs in di George syndrome.
    (e) T—Recurrent infections occur in di George syndrome because of the lack of T cells.

20. (a) T—Complement proteins are proenzymes.
    (b) F—Complement can also be activated by lectins, which bind bacteria.
    (c) F—The alternative pathway is activated spontaneously, particularly on cell surfaces.
    (d) T—The MAC is formed from C5, C6, C7, C8 and C9.
    (e) T—C3 convertase provides a major amplification step.

21. (a) F—Antigen enters lymph nodes via lymphatics.
    (b) T—Lymph filters from the outside to the inside of the node.
    (c) T—Lymph nodes provide an environment for T and B cell activation.
    (d) T—Lymphocytes leave the blood through high endothelial vessels.
    (e) F—Lymph circulates passively.

22. (a) T—Pharyngeal tonsils are organized MALT.
    (b) T—The appendix is an organized MALT found in the caecum.
    (c) F—The thymus is a secondary lymphoid organ not associated with the mucosa.
    (d) T—Peyer's patches are organized MALT found throughout the small and large intestine.
    (e) F—Inguinal lymph nodes drain lymph from the lower limbs.

23. (a) T—The thymus is bilobed.
    (b) F—The thymus is normally found in the mediastinum, but can extend into the neck.
    (c) T—Over 95% of T cell precursors undergo apoptosis in the thymus.
    (d) F—Stromal cells support developing thymocytes.
    (e) T—Thymic epithelial cells produce several hormones that are essential for the differentiation and maturation of thymocytes.

24. (a) T—T helper cells are usually CD4$^+$.
    (b) T—T cell help is required to produce antibodies against protein antigens.
    (c) T—Cytokines produced by T cells are important in the adaptive and innate immune responses.
    (d) F—T helper cells express TCRs in order to detect MHC class II molecules and antigen on APCs.
    (e) T—Different T helper subsets mediate antibody or cell-mediated responses.

25. (a) T—Vascular changes and neutrophil infiltration are mediated by several chemical mediators.
    (b) T—TNF-α is one of the important mediators.
    (c) F—Activation of the complement system produces important mediators for acute inflammation.
    (d) T—Coagulation and fibrinolytic systems are also involved in acute inflammation.
    (e) F—ICAM molecules are upregulated on endothelial cells.

26. (a) T—Adhesion molecules are induced on the endothelium.
    (b) T—Production of platelet-activating factor and prostacyclin is increased.
    (c) T—Neutrophils are attracted by chemotactic cytokines.
    (d) T—Fibroblasts proliferate and increase collagen synthesis.
    (e) T—Cytokines are involved in the development of the acute phase response.

27. (a) F—PAF is produced from cell membrane phospholipids but not from arachidonic acid.
    (b) T—Leukotriene B$_4$ is produced from 5-HPETE a metabolite of arachidonic acid.
    (c) T—Thromboxane A$_2$ is an endoperoxide produced from the metabolism of arachidonic acid.
    (d) F—Perforin is produced and stored in vesicles in cytotoxic T cells and natural killer cells.
    (e) T—Prostacyclin is an endoperoxide produced from the metabolism of arachidonic acid.

28. (a) T—Neutrophils are the first cells to sites of inflammation.
    (b) F—L-selectin is constitutively expressed by leucocytes, whereas E- and P-selectin must be induced on endothelial cells.
    (c) T—Integrin molecules are rapidly induced and strengthen binding.
    (d) T—Integrin molecules such as $\alpha_4\beta_7$ are important for leucocyte homing.
    (e) F—Leucocytes change shape to move between endothelial cells.

29. (a) F—Macrophages and not neutrophils dominate chronic inflammation.
    (b) T—Macrophages are central to chronic inflammation.
    (c) T—Granulomas can result as part of a chronic inflammatory process.
    (d) T—TNF-α is needed for granuloma formation and maintenance.
    (e) F—Lymphocytes are always involved in chronic inflammatory responses.

30. (a) T—Tissue injury is caused by release of several mediators including toxic oxygen metabolites.
    (b) F—A chronic inflammatory response will persist or result in scar formation.
    (c) T—Systemic features, such as weight loss and persistent fever, are characteristic features of chronic inflammation.
    (d) T—Macrophages present antigen to T cells.
    (e) T—Macrophages release fibrogenic cytokines.

31. (a) F—Lysozyme is an important part of the innate response to bacteria.
    (b) T—Antibodies can bind to free virus, preventing entry to cells and increasing phagocytosis.
    (c) T—Interferons induce antiviral states in uninfected cells and activate macrophages and natural killer cells.
    (d) F—Eosinophils are involved in the response against large extracellular parasites such as helminths.
    (e) T—Cytotoxic T cells recognize virally infected cells and kill them.

32. (a) T—Some viruses undergo gradual mutation, the new mutant strain causes a fresh epidemic every few years, e.g. influenza.
    (b) T—MHC expression is reduced by several viruses, including CMV, EBV and adenovirus.
    (c) T—Viruses with unstable genomes (e.g. HIV) undergo mutation within the host. The mutated viruses escape the immune system.
    (d) F—Some bacteria release exotoxins. Viral genomes are too small to encode exotoxins.
    (e) T—HSV, EBV and varicella zoster can become latent.

33. (a) T—Antigenic variation circumvents immunological memory.
    (b) T—Trypanosomes and malaria are immunosuppressive.
    (c) T—Protozoa often have several different stages during infection, thereby presenting several challenges to the immune system.
    (d) T—By infecting intracellularly, humoral immunity is less effective.
    (e) T—Trypanosomes can escape from phagosomes into the cytoplasm.

34. (a) F—IgE mediates type I reactions.
    (b) T—Complexes composed of antigen and antibody cause type III hypersensitivity.
    (c) T—Mast cell degranulation causes type I hypersensitivity.
    (d) F—Rhesus incompatibility is a type II hypersensitivity reaction.
    (e) T—In the Arthus reaction, immune complexes are deposited in the tissues.

35. (a) T—The skin-prick test is for type I (allergic) hypersensitivity.
    (b) T—A Mantoux test looks for type IV hypersensitivity against mycobacterium.
    (c) T—Allergic rhinitis is a type I reaction.
    (d) T—Graves' disease is a type II reaction where antibodies stimulate thyroid cell surface TSH receptors.
    (e) F—Rheumatoid arthritis is a hypersensitivity reaction. Osteoarthritis is believed to be a degenerative condition.

36. (a) F—Paracetamol is not a good anti-inflammatory.
    (b) F—Steroids can be given orally or topically as well as intravenously.
    (c) F—NSAIDs inhibit cyclo-oxygenase.
    (d) T—Anti-TNF-α is a new type of anti-inflammatory drug.
    (e) T—Adverse effects of NSAIDs include nephrotoxicity, bronchospasm and gastrointestinal upset.

37. (a) T—Allergies are type I immediate reactions. They can become chronic, in which case, IgE is still involved.
    (b) T—In asthma, airway obstruction can be reversed by 15% or more.
    (c) T—Pollen and dust mites are common allergens.
    (d) T—Atopic conditions include hay fever, asthma and atopic eczema.
    (e) F—Anaphylaxis is associated with hypotension and shock.

38. (a) T—Densensitization consists of controlled exposure to graded doses of allergen.
    (b) F—Antihistamines control the symptoms of allergy but do not cure them.
    (c) T—Steroids are commonly used in asthma and eczema.
    (d) T—Intramuscular or intravenous adrenaline is important for the resuscitation of patients with anaphylaxis.
    (e) T—Many asthmatics can become symptom free by using prophylactic treatment.

39. (a) T—Central tolerance in the bone marrow or thymus deletes the most self-reactive lymphocytes.
    (b) T—Anergic cells do not respond to antigen.
    (c) F—Molecular mimicry can initiate autoimmunity by breaking self tolerance.
    (d) T—Immune privileged sites can express Fas ligand, causing T cells to apoptose and thereby preventing exposure to sequestered antigen.
    (e) T—Regulatory T cells are important for peripheral tolerance.

40. (a) F—SLE is systemic.
    (b) F—SLE occurs nine times more commonly in women than men.
    (c) T—SLE patients produce antibodies which react with anti-double-stranded DNA or ribonucleoproteins.
    (d) F—SLE is associated with HLA-DR2 or DR3.
    (e) T—A photosensitive malar 'butterfly' rash is common.

41. (a) T—RA is characterized by inflammation of the synovium and destruction of the articular cartilage.
    (b) F—Inflammation affects many tissues in RA.
    (c) T—New treatment strategies aim to block the effects of TNF.
    (d) T—RA occurs in three times as many women as men.
    (e) F—The precise autoantigen(s) in RA are not defined.

42. (a) F—25% of people with RA will not be RF positive.
    (b) T—Rheumatoid factor is an autoantibody.
    (c) F—Rheumatoid factor is an IgM antibody directed against IgG.
    (d) T—Complement activation can occur.
    (e) T—Rheumatoid factor amplifies the immune response.

43. (a) F—Reiter's syndrome is a triad of arthritis, conjunctivitis and urethritis.
    (b) T—Hashimoto's thyroiditis is a cause of goitreous hypothyroidism.
    (c) T—Myasthenia gravis results from anti-acetylcholine receptor antibodies.
    (d) T—Graves' disease results from anti-TSH receptor antibodies.
    (e) F—Polyarteritis nodosa is an autoimmune disease affecting the vasculature (vasculitis).

44. (a) T—It is a primary deficiency in neutrophil killing.
    (b) T—Transient hypogammaglobulinaemia of infancy occurs if the production of antibody by infants is delayed or if the baby is born prematurely.
    (c) F—Splenectomy is not a cause of primary immunodeficiency but can result in a predisposition to infection.
    (d) F—AIDS is a secondary immunodeficiency.
    (e) T—Wiskott–Aldrich syndrome produces a primary lymphocyte deficiency.

45. (a) T—Resulting from chronic bronchial infection.
    (b) T—Resulting from chronic gastrointestinal tract infection.
    (c) F—Rheumatoid arthritis is not associated with antibody deficiency.
    (d) F—Antibody deficiency reduces viscosity.
    (e) T—Mycoplasma is common in antibody deficiency.

46. (a) T—B cells are polyclonally activated in HIV infection.
    (b) T—T cells become defective.
    (c) F—Viral replication can be high even during the latent phase of HIV infection.
    (d) T—Antibodies are generated against gp120 and gp41 but they are not effective at clearing infection.
    (e) T—Lymph nodes become persistently large during HIV infection.

47. (a) T—CMV retinitis occurs at CD4 counts below 50.
    (b) T—*Pneumocystis carinii* pneumonia is common if the CD4 count falls below 200.
    (c) T—Oesophageal candidiasis is common at CD4 counts below 200.
    (d) T—*Mycobacterium avium intracellulare* (MAC) is common at CD4 counts below 50.
    (e) T—Toxoplasmosis is common at CD4 counts below 200.

48. (a) F—MMR is given at 12–15 months and again at 4–5 years.
    (b) T—BCG is given to neonates in at risk groups or at 10–14 years of age. Some countries do not give BCG routinely, e.g. US.
    (c) T—Influenza vaccine is given to at risk groups, including over 65-year-olds.
    (d) T—Meningococcal C vaccine is given at 2, 3 and 4 months.
    (e) T—Tetanus vaccine requires several boosters.

49. (a) T—The Sabin vaccine uses live polio; the Salk vaccine is inactivated polio.
    (b) F—Tetanus toxoid is used for vaccination.
    (c) T—The Bacille Calmette–Guérin vaccine is used for tuberculosis.
    (d) T—Rubella is a live vaccine.
    (e) F—Hepatitis B vaccine uses surface antigen.

50. (a) F—Hyperacute rejection is rapid because antibodies have been induced prior to transplantation, e.g. by blood transfusion.
    (b) F—Acute cellular rejection is mediated by T cells.
    (c) F—Preformed antibodies against HLA cause hyperacute rejection.
    (d) T—Chronic rejection can be caused by deposition of immune complexes, cell-mediated rejection, or viral infection.
    (e) T—The complement and clotting cascades are activated in hyperacute rejection.

51. (a) T—A monozygous twin is genetically identical and should not stimulate the immune system.
    (b) T—Steroids are useful anti-inflammatory and immunosuppressive drugs.
    (c) T—Antibodies to T cells can reduce the risk of transplant rejection.
    (d) T—'Warm ischaemia' is a major risk factor for transplant rejection.
    (e) F—Most transplants are more successful if HLA molecules and blood group antigens are matched.

52. (a) T—Haemopoiesis starts in the bone marrow prior to birth and does not occur elsewhere unless the bone marrow fails to meet the need for new cells.
    (b) T—Bone marrow is found throughout the skeleton.
    (c) T—Yellow bone marrow is almost entirely fat.
    (d) T—Bone marrow macrophages transfer iron to developing red cells, remove debris from haemopoiesis and regulate differentiation and maturation of haemopoietic cells.
    (e) T—T lymphocyte precursors are formed in the bone marrow but move to the thymus for maturation.

53. (a) F—The spleen is posterior to the stomach on the left side of the body.
    (b) T—The red pulp removes old or defective erythrocytes and platelets from the circulation.
    (c) F—Most of the B cell follicles in the spleen will have been stimulated.
    (d) T—The spleen starts developing during the 5th week of fetal life.
    (e) T—Primary cancers of the spleen are very rare.

54. (a) F—Haematopoietic stem cells are found in the liver and spleen, as well as in the bone marrow.
    (b) T—They can differentiate into any of the blood cells.
    (c) T—Stem cells self replicate.
    (d) T—Stem cells divide to become lineage committed stem cells.
    (e) T—The actions of growth factors allow lineage commitment and differentiation.

55. (a) T—Congestive splenomegaly is due to venous congestion.
    (b) F—In the UK, splenomegaly is most commonly due to haematological disorders.
    (c) T—Splenic infarction occurs in myeloproliferative disorders and sickle-cell disease.
    (d) T—EBV infection, trauma and haemopoietic disorders can cause splenic rupture.
    (e) T—The spleen can become enlarged due to lymphomas and leukaemias.

56. (a) T—The spleen is removed to stop blood loss.
    (b) T—Splenic tumours are an indication for splenectomy.
    (c) T—Idiopathic thrombocytopenic purpura can be treated by splenectomy.
    (d) T—Haemolytic anaemias can be improved by splenectomy.
    (e) T—Splenic cysts are an indication for splenectomy.

57. (a) T—Hereditary spherocytosis is an autosomal dominant condition due to inheritance of a defective spectrin gene.
    (b) F—Leads to extravascular haemolysis.
    (c) T—Spherocytes are seen in the peripheral blood.
    (d) T—Spherocytes lyse in less hypotonic solutions than normal red cells.
    (e) F—Spherocytes lyse readily on incubation at 37°C (autohaemolysis).

58. (a) T—In β-thalassaemia major a severe microcytic, hypochromic anaemia is seen.
    (b) T—Iron overload is caused by increased enteric absorption and regular blood transfusions.
    (c) F—Most red blood cells are destroyed in the marrow, those that reach the circulation have a shortened lifespan.
    (d) T—β-thalassaemia major is due to two defective copies of the β-chain gene.
    (e) F—HbA is not present on electrophoresis.

59. (a) F—Erythrocytes are not nucleated.
    (b) T—They are derived from the CFU-GEMM along with granulocytes, macrophages and megakaryocytes.
    (c) T—Their primary function is the transport of O_2 and CO_2.
    (d) F—The normal lifespan is 120 days.
    (e) F—They have a biconcave discoid shape.

60. (a) F—Iron is actively absorbed in the duodenum and jejunum.
    (b) F—There is no mechanism to excrete excess iron.
    (c) F—Iron is transported in the blood bound to transferrin (it is stored with apoferritin).
    (d) T—Primary haemochromatosis is an autosomal recessive disorder characterized by excessive intestinal absorption of iron.
    (e) F—Total body stores of iron are ~4g.

61. (a) F—Adult haemoglobin is composed of two α chains with either two β, or two δ chains.
    (b) T—Oxygen is transported by haemoglobin bound to haem.
    (c) T—Increased H^+ concentration causes the oxygen dissociation curve to shift to the right, the Bohr effect.
    (d) T—Oxygen binding follows a sigmoidal curve, due to allosteric interactions between the subunits.
    (e) F—2,3-diphosphoglycerate levels rise during hypoxia to increase the release of oxygen at the tissues.

62. (a) F—Vitamin B_{12} is absorbed in the terminal ileum after combining with intrinsic factor produced in the stomach.
    (b) T—It is composed of colalamin (cobalt containing) bound to a methyl or adenosyl group.
    (c) T—Absorption is reduced after total gastrectomy due to a lack of intrinsic factor.
    (d) F—Requires intrinsic factor for absorption.
    (e) F—It cannot be synthesized by the body.

63. (a) T—Folic acid is found primarily in green vegetables.
    (b) F—Folic acid is absorbed in the duodenum and jejunum.
    (c) F—The daily requirement is 100–200μg.
    (d) T—Deficiency can be caused by malabsorption in coeliac disease.
    (e) F—During pregnancy, folic acid requirement is increased, and supplements are often given to prevent neural tube defects in the fetus.

64. (a) F—Iron deficiency causes a microcytic anaemia.
    (b) T—Tuberculosis causes a normochromic, normocytic anaemia of chronic disease.
    (c) T—Rheumatoid arthritis causes a normochromic, normocytic anaemia of chronic disease.
    (d) F—Vitamin B_{12} causes a macrocytic anaemia.
    (e) F—Thalassaemia causes a microcytic anaemia.

65. (a) T—Glossitis is a feature of iron-deficiency anaemia.
    (b) T—Koilonychia is a feature specific to iron-deficiency anaemia.
    (c) F—The anaemia produced is microcytic.
    (d) T—It is distinguished from thalassaemia and anaemia of chronic disease by a low serum iron and ferritin.
    (e) F—Serum transferrin is increased in iron deficiency.

66. (a) T—Polycythaemia rubra vera is a primary cause of polycythaemia.
    (b) F—Dehydration causes a relative polycythaemia.
    (c) T—Renal carcinoma causes an absolute polycythaemia due to increased erythropoietin.
    (d) T—Cyanotic heart disease causes an absolute polycythaemia due to increased erythropoietin.
    (e) F—Diuretic therapy causes a relative polycythaemia.

67. (a) T—Pronormoblasts are erythrocyte precursors.
    (b) T—Normoblasts are erythrocyte precursors.
    (c) F—Stomatocytes are seen in liver disease and in alcoholism.
    (d) T—Reticulocytes are erythrocyte precursors.
    (e) F—Echinocytes are seen in renal disease.

68. (a) T—Pigment gallstones are due to excess bilirubin from the breakdown of protoporphyrin.
    (b) F—Plasma haptoglobin falls because it binds to the free haemoglobin in the blood.
    (c) T—Haemosiderin is excreted in the urine.
    (d) T—Release of haemoglobin from lysed erythrocytes.
    (e) T—Excess reticulocytes enter the blood in an effort to increase red cell mass.

69. (a) T—Infection is an oxidizing factor associated with haemolysis when there is a lack of reduced glutathione.
    (b) F—Acidosis, e.g. diabetic ketoacidosis, precipitates haemolysis.
    (c) T—Primaquine is an oxidizing factor associated with haemolysis when there is a lack of reduced glutathione.
    (d) T—Fava beans are oxidizing factors associated with haemolysis when there is a lack of reduced glutathione.
    (e) F—The circulation should be supported during an acute crisis.

70. (a) T—Pneumococcal, meningococcal and Hib vaccine are routinely given to patients with sickle-cell anaemia.
    (b) T—Folic acid is given due to an increased rate of erythropoiesis.
    (c) T—Penicillin prophylaxis and antibiotics for prompt treatment of infections are commonly used.
    (d) T—Blood or exchange transfusions can be given to maintain an adequate haemoglobin level.
    (e) T—Fluids are often needed in the management of acute crises.

71. (a) T—It has a sigmoidal oxygen dissociation curve.
    (b) F—Has a higher affinity for oxygen than adult haemoglobin.
    (c) T—It may persist in β-thalassaemia, to increase the oxygen carrying capacity of blood.
    (d) T—It is produced in the fetal liver and spleen.
    (e) F—Fetal haemoglobin is composed of two α and two γ chains.

72. (a) T—Erythropoietin is required for red-cell maturation, where it prevents red-cell precursors from undergoing apoptosis.
    (b) F—The kidneys are the principle source of erythropoietin.
    (c) T—The major stimulus for release is hypoxia.
    (d) T—Recombinant erythropoietin is indicated for use in a number of clinical diseases.
    (e) F—Required for red-cell maturation.

73. (a) T—It can be caused by drugs, irradiation and chemicals. 50% are idiopathic.
    (b) T—It may be part of a congenital syndrome.
    (c) T—It may be associated with acute viral infection.
    (d) F—Aplastic anaemia is a pancytopenia resulting from aplastic bone marrow.
    (e) T—Androgens are used to treat aplastic anaemia.

74. (a) T—Prosthetic heart valves can cause fragmentation of red cells.
    (b) T—Acute renal failure is a feature of intravascular haemolysis.
    (c) F—Bilirubin is not found in urine because it is bound to albumin.
    (d) T—Increased urobilinogen is common.
    (e) F—The anaemia is normo- or macrocytic.

75. (a) F—Polymorphonuclear leucocytes (neutrophils) have a multilobed nucleus.
    (b) F—They respond primarily to bacterial infection.
    (c) T—They have a granular cytoplasm.
    (d) T—They are phagocytic.
    (e) T—They are a major constituent of pus.

76. (a) T—Myelodysplastic syndromes are acquired bone marrow neoplasias.
    (b) F—Are due to defects in myeloid precursors.
    (c) T—They slowly progress to acute myeloid leukaemia.
    (d) F—Most commonly occur in elderly men.
    (e) T—Prognosis is worst in those with high levels of marrow blasts (>5%).

77. (a) T—Leucostatic symptoms occur in leukaemias.
    (b) F—They are caused by white-cell thrombi.
    (c) T—They do include retinal haemorrhage.
    (d) T—They do include reduced level of consciousness.
    (e) F—They resolve if the white-cell count decreases.

78. (a) T—Superficial, asymmetric, painless lymphadenopathy is consistent with a diagnosis of non-Hodgkin's lymphoma.
    (b) F—Reed–Sternberg cells are pathognomonic of Hodgkin's disease.
    (c) T—Fever, night sweats and weight loss are all features of non-Hodgkin's lymphoma.
    (d) T—Non-Hodgkin's lymphoma is associated with inherited disorders such as Fanconi's syndrome.
    (e) T—Non-Hodgkin's lymphoma is associated with immunodeficiency, e.g. HIV or immunosuppressive therapy.

79. (a) T—Polycythaemia rubra vera is a myeloproliferative disorder.
    (b) F—Sideroblastic anaemia is a myelodysplastic syndrome.
    (c) T—Myelofibrosis is a myeloproliferative disorder.
    (d) T—Primary thrombocythaemia is a myeloproliferative disorder.
    (e) F—Acute lymphoblastic leukaemia is a disease of lymphoid not myeloid lineage.

80. (a) T—Macrophages are differentiated monocytes found in the tissues.
    (b) T—Their primary roles include phagocytosis.
    (c) T—They play an important role in the adaptive immune response.
    (d) T—They may be infected by HIV.
    (e) F—Macrophages are not important in allergic responses (mast cells).

81. (a) T—Chronic lymphocytic leukaemia accounts for 20–50% of leukaemias.
    (b) F—And is a slowly progressing condition.
    (c) T—95% are B cell in origin.
    (d) T—Autoimmune haemolytic anaemias are common.
    (e) F—It never converts to an acute leukaemia.

82. (a) T—Acute lymphoblastic leukaemia is the most common leukaemia in childhood and is rare in adults.
    (b) T—The best prognosis is between the ages of 2 and 10.
    (c) F—Remission rates of over 70% are seen.
    (d) F—80% of cases are B cell in origin.
    (e) T—Aetiological factors include radiation, chemicals, Down syndrome and Fanconi's syndrome.

83. (a) F—Acute myeloblastic leukaemia is an accumulation of primitive myeloblasts in the bone marrow and peripheral blood.
    (b) T—It is associated with hereditary abnormalities such as Down syndrome.
    (c) F—It can be due to a variety of chromosomal rearrangements (isochromosome 12p is associated with testicular tumours).
    (d) F—Only 15% of over-60-year-olds are cured.
    (e) T—Patients are often unwell at presentation and can have a bleeding disorder.

84. (a) T—Chronic myeloid leukaemia is usually identified in the chronic phase, either incidentally or due to constitutional or leucostatic symptoms.
    (b) F—>90% of patients progress to an accelerated phase or blast crisis within 10 years.
    (c) T—The Philadelphia chromosome t(9;22) is identified in more than 90% of cases.
    (d) T—The Philadelphia chromosome is the target for the tyrosine kinase inhibitor Glivec.
    (e) T—Bone marrow transplantation is potentially curative but is not commonly used.

85. (a) F—Monoclonal light chains are produced in a large quantity and are excreted in urine, where they are known as Bence-Jones protein.
    (b) T—Neurological lesions occur due to vertebral collapse.
    (c) T—An acquired hypogammaglobulinaemia and neutropenia leads to repeated infection.
    (d) T—It causes multiple osteolytic bone lesions.
    (e) T—Multiple myeloma is a malignant proliferation of plasma cells, which make up more than 10% of bone marrow cells.

86. (a) T—Aplastic anaemia is a cause of generalized marrow failure.
    (b) T—Leukaemia is also a cause of generalized marrow failure.
    (c) T—Kostmann's syndrome is a congenital defect resulting in neutropenia.
    (d) T—Causes generalized marrow suppression.
    (e) T—Several different drugs, including chloroquine, can lead to a neutropenia.

87. (a) F—Platelets are derived from megakaryocyte cytoplasm.
    (b) F—Platelet adhesion or aggregation requires von Willebrand's factor.
    (c) T—They form a primary platelet plug to slow bleeding.
    (d) T—Platelets interact with type I, II and III collagen via GPIa.
    (e) F—Aggregation is enhanced by thromboxane A_2 and inhibited by prostacyclin.

88. (a) T—Many drugs can cause increased bleeding including marrow suppressants and anticoagulants.
    (b) T—Chemo- and radiotherapy cause bleeding by damage to tissues and reduction in platelets due to marrow suppression.
    (c) T—Haemophila A and B are X-linked.
    (d) T—Splenomegaly leads to increased sequestration and destruction of platelets.
    (e) T—Defective platelets cannot form the primary haemostatic plug.

89. (a) T—Factor II (prothrombin) is a vitamin-K-dependent clotting factor.
    (b) T—Factor IX is a vitamin-K-dependent clotting factor.
    (c) F—Vitamin K acts by allowing post-translational γ-carboxylation of glutamic acid residues.
    (d) T—It is a fat-soluble vitamin and deficiency can result from fat malabsorption.
    (e) F—Haemophilia A is caused by a factor VIII deficiency.

90. (a) T—The prothrombin time is increased in disseminated intravascular coagulation.
    (b) F—In von Willebrand's disease bleeding time is extended and activated partial thromboplastin time may be prolonged.
    (c) T—The prothrombin time is increased in vitamin K deficiency.
    (d) F—Activated partial thromboplastin time is increased in haemophila A but the prothrombin time is normal.
    (e) F—Activated partial thromboplastin time is increased in haemophila B but the prothrombin time is normal.

91. (a) T—Factor V Leiden is less sensitive to inactivation by protein C and therefore confers an increased risk of clotting.
    (b) T—Disseminated cancers secrete substances that activate factor X.
    (c) T—Oestrogen therapy increases levels of the vitamin-K-dependent factors and lowers antithromin III and tissue plasminogen activator levels.
    (d) T—Protein C inhibits factors V and VIII and enhances fibrinolysis, therefore a deficiency increases the risk of clotting.
    (e) T—Prolonged immobilization causes venous stasis and clotting.

92. (a) F—Idiopathic thrombocytopenic purpura (ITP) is caused either by antibody–viral-antigen complexes or anti-platelet IgG autoantibodies.
    (b) T—IgG anti-platelet antibodies are found in the plasma
    (c) T—It occurs in disorders causing an aberrant immune response such as HIV disease.
    (d) T—High-dose glucocorticoids are used in ITP to suppress the abnormal immune response.
    (e) F—Fresh-frozen plasma will not raise the platelet count.

93. (a) F—Heparin is given intravenously or subcutaneously.
    (b) F—Standard heparin is monitored by activated partial thromboplastin time (APTT), low-molecular-weight heparin does not need APTT monitoring.
    (c) T—Heparin is a glycosaminoglycan.
    (d) T—At different molecular weights the activity of heparin is different, with lower molecular weight heparins having greater activity against factor Xa than standard heparin.
    (e) F—Heparin (mucopolysaccharide) and warfarin (coumarin or indandione derivatives) are not structurally related.

94. (a) T—Proteins C and S inhibit clotting factors V and VIII and enhance fibrinolysis.
    (b) F—Plasminogen activator inhibitors prevent fibrinolysis by plasmin.
    (c) T—Reduced levels of platelets diminish clotting.
    (d) T—Streptokinase is a fibrinolytic agent.
    (e) F—Christmas factor (factor IX) is part of the coagulation cascade.

95. (a) F—Haemophilia A is X-linked.
    (b) F—Haemophilia A is not associated with social class.
    (c) F—Treated prophylactically with factor VIII.
    (d) T—Repeated bleeds into joints results in deformity.
    (e) T—It is caused by factor VIII deficiency and so may be mimicked by von Willebrand's disease (pseudohaemophilia).

96. (a) T—The normal haemoglobin for a male is 13–17g/dL.
    (b) T—Normal white cell count is $4–10 \times 10^9$/L.
    (c) T—pO_2 is normally 100mmHg in arterial blood, although 40mmHg is the normal level in mixed venous blood.
    (d) F—Reticulocytes should account for only 1–2% of peripheral red blood cells.
    (e) F—Normal platelet levels are $150–400 \times 10^9$/L.

97. (a) T—Howell–Jolly bodies are inclusions in red cells seen on a peripheral blood smear after splenectomy.
    (b) T—Auer rods are inclusions in white cells seen on a peripheral blood smear of a patient with AML.
    (c) F—Philadelphia chromosome is detected by cytogenetic techniques.
    (d) T—Reticulocytosis may be detected.
    (e) F—Bence-Jones protein is found only in urine.

98. (a) F—People who are blood group O can have parents who are both group O, although parents who are heterozygous for group A or B can pass on an O allele.
    (b) T—Group A people will produce anti-B antibodies.
    (c) F—In blood group O it is the H antigen that is left unchanged.
    (d) F—Group AB is the universal recipient and group O the universal donor.
    (e) F—Anti-ABO antibodies are IgM leading to intravascular haemolysis.

99. (a) T—Rhesus D incompatibility is a common cause of haemolytic disease of the newborn.
    (b) F—It doesn't usually occur in the first child because the mother has not been sensitized to the rhesus D antigen before.
    (c) F—Rhesus D is not the only cause of haemolytic disease of the newborn.
    (d) T—Passive immunization can prevent the mother producing antibodies.
    (e) F—The antibodies are IgG.

100. (a) T—Donor red cells are destroyed by IgM antibodies in the recipient's serum.
    (b) T—IgM antibodies can fix complement.
    (c) F—Symptoms occur within minutes to hours.
    (d) F—Hypo- not hypertension occurs, but the other symptoms are present.
    (e) T—Release of tissue thromboplastin from lysed red cells can lead to disseminated intravascular coagulation.

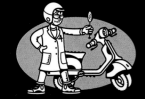

1. Refer to Fig. 1.39, p. 33.

2. Positive and negative selection of T cells occurs during T cell maturation in the thymus. Positive selection of T cells refers to the process whereby T cells that are capable of binding self-major histocompatibility complex (MHC) molecules are selected for. It involves the interaction of developing CD4+ CD8+ T cells with thymic epithelial cells that express high levels of class I and class II molecules. T cells that do not interact with MHC undergo apoptosis. This is because they do not receive a protective signal as a result of the interaction between the T cell receptor (TCR) and MHC.

   Some of the T cells that survive positive selection have receptors with high affinity for self-MHC and self-antigen. These CD4+ CD8+ T cells undergo negative selection. Negative selection is thought to be mediated by dendritic cells (which are derived from the bone marrow). These cells express high levels of class I and class II MHC molecules, which interact with T cells expressing high-affinity receptors for self-MHC alone or self-MHC and antigen. These 'self-reactive' T cells are, therefore, removed via apoptosis.

   The positive and negative selection processes result in a population of thymocytes that can bind self-MHC at low affinity but are not stimulated by self-MHC plus self-antigen. Positive selection occurs in the cortex of the thymus. Negative selection occurs in the corticomedullary junction and medulla of the thymus.

3. Refer to Fig. 4.9, p. 81.

4. The structure of an Ig molecule is shown in Fig. 1.29. The functions are:
   - Complement fixation.
   - Opsonization.
   - Neutralization of toxins.
   - Participation in antibody-dependent cell-mediated cytotoxicity.
   - Protection of the neonate (IgG crossing the placenta and IgA in breast milk).
   - Mast cell activation in parasitic infestations (IgE).

5. Pernicious anaemia is a chronic atrophic gastritis with a probable autoimmune aetiology. It is the most common cause of vitamin B_{12} deficiency in adults. Autoantibodies directed against both the gastric parietal cells and intrinsic factor (IF) are detectable in the serum and gastric juice of most patients. Damage to the parietal cells and failure of formation and absorption of the B_{12}–IF complex result.

   Achlorhydria is an accompanying feature (parietal cells are also responsible for secreting H^+). Pernicious anaemia is associated with autoimmune thyroid disease and patients are at an increased risk of gastric carcinoma. Clinical features include:

- A lemon-yellow colour to the skin, caused by a combination of pallor and jaundice resulting from ineffective erythropoiesis.
- Glossitis.
- Gastrointestinal disturbances.
- Weight loss.
- Neurological abnormalities (peripheral neuropathy, subacute degeneration of the spinal cord involving the posterior and lateral columns, and psychiatric disturbances).

The diagnosis is made by either demonstrating the presence of antibodies to intrinsic factor in the patient's serum or by using the Schilling test.

6. Haemolytic disease of the newborn is the result of the passage of IgG antibodies from the maternal circulation across the placenta into the fetal circulation, where they react with fetal red cells and lead to their destruction by the fetal reticuloendothelial system (RES). Haemolytic disease of the newborn can result when a rhesus-negative woman becomes pregnant with a rhesus-negative fetus. During the first pregnancy, the mother is usually sensitized during childbirth, when small amounts of fetal blood leak into the maternal circulation. The mother mounts an antibody response directed against the rhesus antigens. During subsequent pregnancies with a rhesus-positive fetus, IgG antibodies cross the placenta and bind to fetal red cells, resulting in haemolysis. Most cases are due to anti-D antibodies. The most severe consequence is hydrops fetalis.

   Prevention is by intramuscular administration of anti-D IgG to the rhesus-negative mother at 28 weeks and within 72 hours of birth. The D surface antigen on fetal red blood cells in the maternal circulation is coated, thereby preventing a maternal immune response. The rhesus-positive red-blood-cell–anti-D-antibody complex is then removed in the maternal RES.

   Haemolytic disease of the newborn can also be caused by other red blood cell incompatibilities, e.g. Kell or Duffy antigens.

7. Innate immunity comprises the non-specific mechanisms that exist prior to exposure to antigen and are not altered on repeated exposure to a particular antigen. The immune system provides a rapid, non-specific response.

   Adaptive immunity is characterized by specificity and memory. Specificity refers to the ability of the adaptive immune response to distinguish minor differences between antigens. Memory refers to the fact that, once the adaptive immune system has responded to an antigen, it responds more rapidly and to a greater degree upon subsequent exposures, but is still slower than the innate system.

An antigen is any molecule that can be recognized by the adaptive immune system.

An immunogen is a molecule that evokes an immune response. All immunogens are antigenic, but not all antigens are immunogenic.

A hapten is a small antigen that is not immunogenic unless coupled to a larger (usually protein) carrier molecule.

An epitope antigenic determinant (or immunologically active portion of antigen) is the discrete area of the antigen that is recognized by the adaptive immune system.

8. Refer to Fig. 2.33, p. 62.

9. Factors II, VII, IX and X, and proteins C and S are dependent on vitamin K for post-translational modification (see Fig. 6.11, p. 122).

Vitamin K acts as a cofactor for the carboxylase enzyme, resulting in γ-carboxylation of glutamic acid residues, enabling them to bind calcium and, therefore, form complexes with the platelet phospholipid membrane.

In the absence of vitamin K, factors II, VII, IX and X do not undergo γ-carboxylation, cannot bind calcium and are unable to attach onto platelet phospholipid membranes. Consequently, they are activated much more slowly and negligible levels of prothrombin are converted to thrombin.

10. Refer to Fig. 6.1 (p. 116) to answer this question.

11. (i) Tuberculosis complicating HIV infection.
    (ii) The finding may have been incidental e.g. when donating blood, or a person who is at risk e.g. intravenous drug abuser or sex worker, may have sought an HIV test. In both cases the person may be asymptomatic or have had a mild flu-like illness. Other presenting features may include: skin – molluscum contagiosum; mouth – oral hairy leucoplakia, oral candidiasis, Kaposi's sarcoma; haematological – immune-mediated thrombocytopenic purpura; infections – meningitis (cryptococcal), pneumonia, sinusitis, recurrent gastrointestinal infections (*Salmonella*, *Cryptosporidium*, *isospora belli*).
    (iii) The underlying condition can be treated with antiretrovirals. They can act at different points within the viral lifecycle.

12. (i) Chronic lymphocytic leukaemia.
    (ii) Demonstrate the classical immunophenotypic features of the blood lymphocytes.
    (iii) Because the disease is slowly progressive and of a low grade, chemotherapy or stem cell therapy are used to limit rather than cure the disease. The median survival is 5–8 years.

13. (i) Multiple myeloma.
    (ii) • Normochromic normocytic anaemia, resulting from marrow infiltration.
        • Repeated infections. These can occur due to hypogammaglobulinaemia and neutropenia.

• Hypercalcaemia, which occurs in 10% of cases. This is due to increased reabsorption of bone and is indicative of advanced disease.
• Chronic renal failure, which occurs in 20–30% of patients. Factors that can contribute to renal failure in multiple myeloma are:
  – increased blood viscosity
  – hypercalcaemia
  – renal tubular obstruction by proteinaceous casts
  – toxic effect of Bence-Jones protein on proximal renal tubules
  – infection
  – dehydration
  – non-steroidal anti-inflammatory drugs
  – light-chain deposition in glomeruli.
• Amyloidosis. This can lead to nephrotic syndrome. An abnormal bleeding tendency occurs owing to the adverse effect of paraprotein on platelets and to coagulation factors.

14. (i) Antibody deficiency.
    (ii) Replacement immunoglobulin in the form of pooled human immunoglobulin.

15. Following splenectomy, the patient should be encouraged to mobilize as soon as possible because he is at high risk of thrombosis. He should be made aware that he will have a lifelong increased risk of infection, particularly from encapsulated organisms, e.g. *Neisseria meningitides*, *Streptococcus pneumoniae*, *Haemophilus influenzae*. The following steps should be taken:
• Pneumococcal vaccine should be given, with boosters every 5–10 years.
• Hib and meningococcal vaccine should also be given.
• Prophylactic antibiotics (penicillin) should be given for life.
• He should be given antibiotics that he must take immediately if any symptoms of infection develop.
• He should be warned that tropical infections, e.g. malaria, are more likely to be severe.
• Urgent hospital admission if infection develops.

16. (i) Open lung biopsy. This diagnostic test aims to make a histological diagnosis.
    (ii) Lymphoma, diffuse carcinoma. This patient had a B cell lymphoma.

17. (i) Concentrated factor VIII or IX (depending on the type of haemophilia), fresh-frozen plasma or blood (if severe blood loss).
    (ii) Acute HIV seroconversion.

In the UK, blood products are now routinely tested for HIV antibodies but this might not be the case in developing countries.

18. (i) Favism.
    (ii) Negative bilirubin, high urobilinogen and positive haemoglobin (strongly positive for blood with no red cells seen on microscopy).
    (iii) Reduced haemoglobin (which might be very low, e.g. 4g/dL) and increased unconjugated bilirubin. Characteristic blood film changes.

19. (i) A full blood count to ascertain the haemoglobin level in view of the ruddy complexion. In addition, you wish to know the white-cell count and platelet count.
    (ii) Exclude secondary reasons for a raised haemoglobin, e.g. hypoxia. Confirm an increase in red cell mass and demonstrate the characteristic bone marrow and clinical features of PRV.
    (iii) Venesection to reduce blood viscosity. May need the use of cytotoxic therapy, e.g. hydroxyurea.

20. (i) Anaphylactic response to the bee sting.
    (ii) The initial management of anaphylaxis is that of resuscitation (airway, breathing, circulation). Adrenaline (epinephrine) should be given intramuscularly and repeated after 5 minutes if there is no improvement. Adrenaline can be given intravenously in life-threatening profound shock or airway obstruction. Fluids might be needed if he is in shock and a β_2-adrenreceptor agonist can be used to reverse bronchospasm. He should be given adrenaline (epipen) to carry with him, so that it can be administered rapidly in an emergency. He should also have a medic alert bracelet. He may undergo venom desensitization.

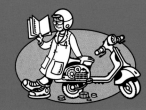

Index